Staying Afloat in a Sea of Forgetfulness

COMMON SENSE CAREGIVING

EXPANDED EDITION

Gary Joseph LeBlanc

To order additional copies of this book, contact:
Xlibris Corporation
1-888-795-4274
www.Xlibris.com
Orders@Xlibris.com
94179

Contents

Acknowledgments

I would like to give endless thanks to all the readers of my column "Common Sense Caregiving" and for all the encouragement I received to take this collection of my articles and compile them into a book.

Also kudos to Duane Chichester and Paula Nelson of the *Hernando Today*. Thank you for believing in me and my work and for running my column and giving me the chance to help my fellow caregivers in the community and also readers miles and miles away.

Additional special thanks need to be given to Holly Beth Michaels and to Faye Verstraete for their patience with my writing; to Fred Mannarino for donating his artistic work creating the front cover; and to Peter Hanen, Esther Marie Latz, Valerie Esker and Gail Teachworth for their generous donations in poetry.

Semper Fi

What I admire most about the Latin motto "*Semper Fidelis*" is that it literally means "Always Faithful"—not just sometimes or just once in a while but *always!* If you are to be a successful and effective caregiver for someone with Alzheimer's, you should make this a truism to live by.

I am as guilty as anyone of commencing to undertake a pursuit and leaving it only half completed. Caregiving is not a science project or any other sort of enterprise. Rather, it's a truly noble campaign with the welfare of our loved ones at stake.

The Alzheimer's disease demands that we pledge to stay adamant and continue to be steadfast by their sides until they exhale their last breath.

Yes, *Semper Fidelis* should become a way of life, not just a fancy slogan. Be proud of what you're doing. Always be faithful to your loved ones. Beware that very few can handle this pilgrimage. This makes you special.

So to my fellow caregivers—if I had a glass in my hand, I would raise it high and propose a toast to you, crying out in highest volume: *"Semper Fidelis!"*

The Characteristics of a Successful Alzheimer's Caregiver

When caring for someone who is suffering from Alzheimer's or dementia, be prepared to face hardships unlike anything you have encountered before. Unfortunately, not everyone who attempts caregiving will be successful.

There's no shame in admitting defeat or the need for help. This ordeal is unequal to any other and if you find that you're suddenly unable to carry out this crusade, please don't go through the rest of your life inflamed with guilt. This is definitely not what your loved one would have wished upon you.

Here are five main characteristics you should try to embrace while fulfilling the role of caregiver. As long as you maintain these significant qualities, you should survive this noble campaign just fine:

Commitment—faithful dedication to the cause of the
  patient until his or her final breath.

You must stay devoted to the very end. Even if there
comes a time when you can no longer care for your
loved one at home and have to place him or her in
a facility, your job is still not finished. You must continue to remain vigilant, constantly making sure their
best interest is always being looked after.

Compassion—concern toward the suffering and
  understanding the feelings of the patient and the
  family members.

One thing that I've learned is that denial is one
symptom of Alzheimer's which affects everyone close
to the patient. Many families are torn apart, some
never healing their wounds. Watching a spouse, parent or sibling dissolve right in front of your eyes is a
devastating experience. So when caring for such an
individual, you must continue to be compassionate
to all that are near. I've talked with many caregivers
who feel straight-out rage toward their relatives for
not assisting in anyway at all. Even as hard as it may
be, please try to put your bitterness aside for the
sake of your loved one. I have learned that patients
tend to feed off emotions. Hostile feelings being
displayed will make the situation more difficult for
both of you.

Endurance—withstanding painful long years of
  misery in defense of the victim and caregiver of
  this dreadful disease.

You have to reach deep inside yourself and pull out all the endurance you can find. It is in there, believe me. Sadly, there is no set time frame for this malady. There have been some cases where victims have suffered a tormenting twenty years with this illness. This is not the norm; they usually only survive six to eight years after they have been diagnosed. But you just never know. So strap your boots on tight and dig your heels in and be prepared for a long haul of asperity.

Unselfishness—generosity of putting your life on hold, including social isolation and financial burdens.

One of the first things you notice when you become a caregiver is that your social life will start withering away. Also most caregivers will have to terminate their employment and in today's economy that is quite troublesome. There are numerous sacrifices that must be made in order to keep your loved one safe and comfortable. Being selfish is something a caregiver simply doesn't even have time for.

Honesty—loyalty toward and the protection of the afflicted one's assets and best interest.

The person you are caring for has placed all the trust they possess in you. Strive to preserve all of their holdings the best you can. You never know what unexpected monetary expenditures will present themselves toward the end of this disease. Thirty-five to forty percent of elder abuse comes from some type of financial devastation.

Stay true to your heart and always follow what instincts that are deep inside. You will know what the right thing is to do. And by trying to follow these five characteristics, you will undoubtedly become a stronger individual.

I realize that maintaining all five of these characteristics will be almost an impossible goal. Just try to abide by as many of them as possible.

Someday, after this arduous campaign is over, you'll be able to look back and know that from this experience you have developed morally and ethically into a better person.

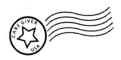

Dear Caregiver,

Throughout this book, I will be preaching continuously of the importance of routine. I learned that it is such a significant issue that it may make or break you as a caregiver.

As Mark Twain once wrote: "Habit is habit, and not to be flung out the window by any man."

GJL

Keeping It Simple

(Routine, Routine, Routine)

Round-the-clock living and taking care of an Alzheimer's patient over the past eight years have unearthed several absolutes for being a caregiver. I do not possess a medical degree, but speak purely from experience; over ten years ago, my father was diagnosed with Alzheimer's disease.

At the very top of the list is routine—a steady, run-of-the-mill lifestyle. In fact, routine is probably wholesome for everybody. It might be boring at times, but if you lack short-term memory, it will be your greatest friend. A habitual life will ease most anxiety and frustration. For instance, I tried to serve Dad's breakfast and dinner at the same time every day; I even used a particular plate for his pills every morning and evening. When I did not, we had a problem: "These aren't the pills I took yesterday." Every day I arranged his silverware in a consistent pattern. Pasta or other food that didn't require a knife still had one placed next to it.

The same applied to clothing. There was no reason for him to make too many choices. Having only three or four outfits kept things uncomplicated. An enchanting young woman once told him how good he looked in red. Well, red it was; for almost a whole year the man wore only red shirts. Funny how certain thoughts lingered inside of his head while others would disappear within seconds. I had to buy four red shirts just so laundry wouldn't have to be done daily. Red pants however, were completely out of the question, thank goodness!

What many people don't realize is that even just a casual trip to the doctor left Dad confused for days. Even so, every two months we visited the same waiting room, with him religiously asking, "Have we ever been here before?" By the time we were home, he could not be convinced that he ever went. The next day, he was completely out of sync. He'd wake up earlier than usual, swearing he never ate in the morning, claiming that he already swallowed his pills, at times becoming straight-out delusional. This may sound minor, but these things have a way of snowballing. By day's end, he was a complete mess. Unfortunately, the chances were that I'd be right there with him.

One day, Dad had two different doctor visits scheduled. This was a variation on an already distressing theme. On the way home he kept insisting that I was going the wrong way, while continuously opening the door as the car was moving!

The easier that life is for your patient, the more pleasant yours will be. I don't imagine this advice will turn up in *The New England Journal of Medicine;* I'm just speaking from what I learned through my own care-giving experience.

You still might have to step outside and kick some dirt around now and then, just to deal with the frustrations. Repeating yourself fifty times a day, answering the same questions over and over and listening to multiple excuses tends to wear the fabric a bit thin.

There always was a superficial excuse for something Dad forgot or why he didn't recognize someone. Here's an example: an emergency room doctor was asking him basic questions to assess his lucidity. One of the questions happened to be, "Do you know who the president is?" He looked at me, then around the room, and said absolutely nothing. The doctor left the room and closed the curtain. Dad promptly quipped, "This guy calls himself a doctor and he doesn't even know who the president is." We could hear the doctor laughing on the other side of that thin curtain wall.

Well, your neighbors might wonder why you're walking in circles, beating up your lawn. Ignore them. Just keep telling yourself, "It's not your loved one's fault"—because it's not. Keep these beloved victims' lives as uncomplicated as possible. Love them and be their most forbearing friend and enjoy them for as long as you still can.

It will be well worth it in the long run.

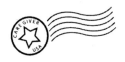

Dear Caregiver,

Each day, as you overcome yet another hurdle, pause and marvel at the strength that is blossoming within you.

Dale Carnegie wrote: "Don't be afraid to give your best to what seemingly are small jobs. Every time you conquer one, it makes you that much stronger. If you do the little jobs well, the big ones tend to take care of themselves."

HBM

Endurance

(Finding Inner Strength and Making Social Sacrifices)

If you're on pins and needles because of worry, stop it! You will always question yourself. Caregivers will forever panic about whether the job they're doing is adequate. Learn from your mistakes; this is not a science. Patients vary from one to another.

Taking care of a memory-impaired person is exhausting and emotionally draining. You'll know when you're about to hit the wall. Don't argue with yourself. Instead find a way to take a break or everything will start to overwhelm you. When you get a chance to get away, go, but try not to spend too much time alone. When I had time to escape, one of my main goals was to refrain from repeating myself thirty times a night. I looked for normal conversation, in which I was not required to answer the same question more than twice.

Caregivers will experience a dwindling effect on their social life. Because of my own school of hard knocks, I can tell you that my telephone practically stopped ringing. I was at the point where I was about to call "Ma Bell" to find out if I was having technical difficulties.

Be advised that friends from the past will eventually stop calling after their invitations to attend gatherings or evenings at the movies have been declined time and time again. Even well-meaning people can be put off by the mere fact that you cannot leave your loved one alone. Recently, a woman said to me, "Nobody realizes that sometimes it's like babysitting a sixteen-armed octopus. You can't leave them alone for a single minute."

The general population has never experienced the 24/7 hardships of caregiving, so naturally they have no conception of the amount of sacrifices that must be made.

While taking care of your loved one, you simply keep telling yourself that your old friends are just on hold. Now that sometime has transpired after my father's passing, I have discovered that only the most sincere and faithful friendships survived.

But, on the other hand, you may find an upside regarding the subject of human relationships and that is the befriending of new acquaintances who are fellow caregivers, people who are walking the same path as you. The support and passion of these strong individuals may be more valuable and emboldening than the companions you knew from your past.

Social isolation is a high-risk factor for developing dementia. This is just one of the reasons for you to remain somewhat socially active. Whether it's through

Internet chat rooms or staying in touch with friends on Facebook, phone calls or even the old fashioned U.S. Mail, it is vital to have some form of communication with the outside world. I highly recommend trying a support group in your area.

When taking care of my father, there would be times when I would suddenly realize that I hadn't left the property in a three-week period. A trip to the barber shop not only becomes a blessing but a major social event!

Learn to cherish the ones that lend you an ear, even if it's only for a couple of minutes. Keep an open mind to the unforeseen new friendships you may encounter. There is something special about socializing with a colleague that is in the same boat as you. Try not to worry about the friends that have slowly slipped away. This demanding journey of caregiving may guide your life into a totally different direction. The endurance and strength required is tremendous. You have to reach deep inside yourself and pull that endurance out. It's in there, believe me.

Fortunately for me, I had a sister who helped me when she was able and constantly told me I was doing a terrific job. If nobody is telling you this, say it to yourself. Heck, yell it out your front door! I'm not going to kid you, this was the hardest thing I ever did in my life, but I wouldn't have had it any other way. But by keeping my dad in a run-of-the-mill routine lifestyle throughout his disease, I was amazed by how well he managed.

You too must guide your loved one through the remainder of his or her life on a simple, beaten path. The sooner you establish this familiar trail, the easier it will be to care for your memory-impaired friend.

Forget about any mistakes you make; everyone makes them. You're better off looking at the humor in the situation; it's there.

Always remember, it's better to laugh than to cry.

Dear Caregiver,

I *always loved the character that Red Skelton played,*"Freddie *the Freeloader."It makes me chuckle just thinking of him. A great line that came from this classic comedian, which reminds me of short-term memory, is:*"I *don't let old age bother me. There are three signs of old age: Loss of memory*—I *forgot the other two."*

GJL

Warning Signs

(Early Symptoms of Alzheimer's)

If you're thinking that it's Friday when it's only Monday, don't panic. This is not a reason to suspect that you're exhibiting signs of Alzheimer's. Most everyone drifts through spells of forgetfulness.

However, if you're worried about yourself or a loved one, there are several warning signs to watch out for. In the initial stages, you might notice that the person begins forgetting things like the following:

- Important dates
- Appointments
- Familiar names

Or the person is starting to show certain characteristics as follows:

- Repeatedly asking the same question
- Having a shorter attention span
- Losing sense of time

Some patients manifest problems working with numbers, such as being unable to balance a checkbook. They may even scribble a check with the date off by decades. Such lapses might appear to be simple mistakes made by someone merely overtired, but when such blunders occur frequently that may be a signal for concern.

Difficulty with reading may also send up a red flag. When the person you're concerned about never makes it off the front page of the newspaper or farther than the first chapter of a book, this will likely point to a possible early loss of attention span.

When your loved ones' condition worsens, excuses will flow like a raging river. Alzheimer's patients become amazingly clever at fabricating excuses. Perhaps you'll think that he or she is just being stubborn, refusing to perform even simple tasks. Remember, it is less embarrassing for them to just say "No" than to appear foolish.

Next come the accusations. When they misplace an item, you or somebody else will undoubtedly be blamed. They could be experiencing swift mood changes or frustration expressed over a simple task or errand.

Often, faltering and struggling for words will emerge later as the disease advances. Patients may no longer join in conversations or even stop speaking in mid-sentence. You can almost see their gears turning, searching to find a common word. My father often called things by the wrong name like, "Please turn up the radio," when in reality he meant the television.

These are changes you need to begin writing down so you can communicate them to the patient's physician. If the diagnosis is to be Alzheimer's, the sooner you know the better. Immediately start to create a plan with family members or assistants who are available.

Please be aware that many of these symptoms could be caused by medications, stress or even depression. This is the reason that it is vitally important that at the onset itself, have your patient given a thorough medical examination.

Hopefully, the diagnosis won't be anything significant and they will be able to enjoy the "golden years" the way they were meant to be spent.

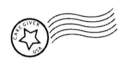

Dear Caregiver,

The daily experience of watching your loved one dissipate is one of the more arduous aspects of caregiving.

H. P. Lovecraft said: "The most merciful thing in the world, I think, is the inability of the human mind to correlate all its contents."

GJL

Empty Thoughts

(Memory Loss)

Friends and even family members would spend maybe ten minutes in conversation with my dad and walk away being satisfied that he was perfectly fine. Their impression would be that I overexaggerated the whole situation. Have you ever had the wind knocked out of you? Indisputably, that is what it feels like. What they didn't realize is the minute they were out of the door, my father was asking, "Who the heck were those people? What were they trying to sell us?"

Having suffered from Alzheimer's for many years, Dad had reached a point where he had absolutely no short-term memory whatsoever. Everything started for him at that very moment—there was no "before." What was happening at the present time was the only world he lived in.

Unfortunately, his long-term memory started to fade as well. There was a time when he could tell you what color sweater he was wearing on a particular day forty yesteryears ago. On the other hand, I had a conversation with him about his two youngest brothers and he had absolutely no recollection of either. Were it not for a family photo album, he probably would have accused me of lying.

He also had great difficulty recognizing our house where he'd lived for the last eighteen years. Often, he would ask if we ever spent an entire season "in this cabin." I believe he was recalling a small cabin from his boyhood where he and his own father would stay overnight while cutting wood for the winter months. Throughout the progression of the disease, sadly, the long-term memory also starts to deteriorate.

There are certain matters an Alzheimer's patient will put forward that you're better off not questioning. One afternoon, Dad kept going on how he remembered my sister at the age of fourteen and how she loved to sit on the swing chair in the front yard and was simultaneously running an auction house. Hardly! The fact of the matter was at that time, she was already the mother of three children and approaching her thirties.

While watching a football game being played in Green Bay, Wisconsin, we noticed the weather there deteriorating into blizzard conditions. Turning his head from the television screen, he told me to call in the cat before she froze to death. Bear in mind—we lived in hot, sunny Florida.

There is one inevitable incident that crumbles every Alzheimer's caregiver. Dad finally asked me who I was. It had already happened with my sisters, mother, and practically everybody else he knew, but this was my first. No smite by the remorseless *"mental invader"* is more atrocious. I felt completely devastated as Dad was altogether stolen away from me. Alas, though I'd been with him since the madness began and tried to prepare myself for that, it came on me like a locomotive steaming down a mountain pass.

In conclusion, I really don't know if there is anything I can do to make the road smoother for you when this happens. And it will. What I can tell you though is that you'll never *really* be forgotten. The disease of Alzheimer's prevents its victims from retrieving their memory at certain times only. You might leave the room, return a minute later and they're glad to see you. Their love for you never really disappears. They just can't retrieve it at certain innocent moments.

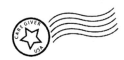

Dear Caregiver,

Lennon and McCartney penned a haunting song in the 1960's "Nowhere Man."

Many times I've gazed upon the confused face and empty eyes of an Alzheimer's patient and remembered the verse "He's a real nowhere man, sitting in his nowhere land, making all his nowhere plans for nobody." Sad isn't it? But this is where you, the caregiver, come on the scene to lift your loved ones' spirits! Love, listen and learn. And remember those all important validating hugs!

HBM

Use It or Lose It

(Staying Mentally Active)

Three thousand days plus—that's how long my father fought his way through the perplexing and demeaning stages of Alzheimer's.

He did extremely well for himself, probably better than most. I truly believe it was from setting the ground rules from the onset, making sure he had a tranquil and routine life, keeping confusion as far away from him as possible.

Limiting bedrock choices and decision-making will help minimize most nervousness and frustration. This holds true even in setting a schedule for meals or daily walks. Once again I am going to emphasize what an important role routine plays in pacifying those who suffer from memory impairment.

Let me again state that my knowledge does not come from a medical diploma. It has been acquired strictly from sharing the woes and burdens of a day-by-day, year-by-year journey, during which it became necessary to draw from my common sense, and the love in my heart to guide me along the way.

In dealing with the devastating changes this cruel disease extorts, I believe one of the most merciless junctures was watching Dad lose control of his attention span. Initially, I noticed things such as his reading of the first three pages of a book several times over or losing patience during television programs. Progression of the disease was characterized by obnoxious verbal and hand gestures toward the boob tube and high decibels of, "You call this acting?" It wasn't so long ago; he had favored such mystery shows as, *Murder She Wrote* or *Hercule Poirot* by Agatha Christie. The relentless progression of Alzheimer's had extinguished all of his short-term memory and convinced him they were all a bunch of idiots. Once a commercial broke, he forever lost track of who murdered whom.

Fortunately, we lived near the Tampa Bay area of Florida's Gulf Coast, where the Tampa Bay Rays had finally turned into a winning major league baseball team. Dad was so much better watching sports. The top of the screen held an attention-getting scoreboard. He would still ask me thirty to fifty times—who's playing or who's winning, but the air traffic flow of four-letter words flying around our living room had diminished immensely.

During his earlier stages, I left the Game Show channel on most of the day. Even when he regressed to scarcely knowing the answers, I'm convinced that those shows kept his upper gears shifting. If he said the answer was blue and they said it was white, next came: "I told you it was white!" Poor Regis Philbin would be quickly dispatched with "This game is rigged!"

Have you ever heard the expression "use it or lose it?" Well, that's where I'm headed with this. Dad played two to three hours of *solitaire* on a daily basis. Sometime back during a moment of clarity, he explained to me that when he played cards, it created some kind of safety bubble for him. I believe that by blocking everything else out, he was able to evade most frustrations and jitteriness for a short period of time. I must tell you that if he wasn't playing cards, I would have been constantly worrying about what else he might have gotten himself into. That safety bubble covered quite a bit of acreage as a sanctuary for him, and a little breather for me.

It's a long, slow and painful ride for any caregiver. Hopefully, these suggestions will help take out some of the bumps along the way for you.

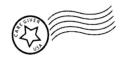

Dear Caregiver,

American poet Maya Angelou wrote: "I've learned that people will forget what you said, people will forget what you did, but people will never forget how you made them feel."

Your loved ones never really forget you. You're still there, deep inside them; they just can't retrieve that memory of you at certain times. But you're always part of them. Trust me.

GJL

Paths to the Past

(Short-Term Memory)

When Dad was first diagnosed with Alzheimer's, a doctor explained to us the difference between long-term and short-term memory loss. This is how he put it, "When you're traveling through the woods to a place you've visited many times, you'll be walking on a trail that will be well broken in. But when you go to a place you've never visited, the brush and branches spring back, devouring the newly made path so you can't find the same way back."

Think of these paths and trails as the highway system of your brain; with childhood memories, you're cruising down a two-lane highway. But when you're trying to think of someone you just met or what just happened two minutes ago, the road you're stumbling upon hasn't even been surveyed and cleared yet.

Dad spoke directly to his physician, "So what you're telling me is I'm going to be lost in the woods forever?"

"No, you'll have many moments of clarity during the first stage of the disease. But as you progress into the middle stage, these moments will find you less and less."

I have to tell you that when my dad would realize all of a sudden he was not where he thought he was, or you're not who he thought you were, the devastation that would spread across his face was heartbreaking. It was one of the saddest parts of watching him deteriorate.

The best thing I found to do was to gently change the subject. I would attempt to move his mind on to something else. Amazingly, his penetrating sadness would usually vaporize as fast as it found him.

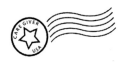

Dear Caregiver,

George William Curtis, writer, public speaker and editor of Harper's Weekly, is known for saying: "It is not the ship so much as the skillful sailing that assures the prosperous voyage."

It's important to use all the skills you learn and maintain your health when you're navigating the course through the storms of caregiving.

GJL

Don't Go Down with the Ship

(Caregiver's Health and Sleeping Habits)

Like a severe tropical storm, being under the weather can shatter a caregiver. You can find yourself in a washout mentally and physically, even taking the strongest of caregivers out for the count. It is imperative to pace yourself and be willing to bear disappointment or you'll find yourself flat on your back, maybe even hospitalized.

Caring for my father, I learned that honoring this obligation can leave you exhausted. Anyone who doesn't realize this hasn't a clue how much self-discipline is involved in caregiving. These are just a few examples:

- Vastly limited social life
- Little or no private time
- Giving up your favorite hobbies
- Unable to attend church services

The list goes on and on.

It is a known fact that stress can kill. Don't let it conquer you. Stand tall. Your health is the key to everything. If you go down, the ship you're navigating will soon become the *Titanic* and head straight to the bottom. Being the primary caregiver means you have to attempt to be indestructible, but remember, that doesn't imply that you have to be a superhero.

Remain consistent with your own doctor visits. I went almost two years without a physician's examination. Look at it as a day out. I know it's not the most enjoyable thing to be doing with your infrequent free time, but at least you'll likely get an hour to yourself while waiting in the examination room.

Also, try to busy yourself with doing something physical for about thirty minutes a day. Maybe some yard work or going for a walk. Try killing two birds with one stone. As for myself, I would mow the grass. It was kind of a sanctuary for me. The grass beneath my kitchen window is trimmed to a neat cemetery-style half inch. This is from cruising by constantly looking in to make sure Dad was still playing solitaire at the dinner table.

If you can't leave your patient alone, place him or her in a lounge chair in the shade. But keep in mind, a trip to the gym is another way of killing two birds with one stone: physical exercise enhanced with some socializing.

One of the most difficult things about caring for someone with Alzheimer's is never really getting a good night's sleep. Have you ever heard the expression "sleeping with one eye open?" Well, it isn't an easy thing to accomplish but, as a caregiver, you may find it necessary to do just that!

I know that when I was caring for my dad, my bed-time consisted of more napping than an actual night's sleep. I would be constantly listening to see if he was moving around, worrying about what chaos he might get himself into. After many years of this, I naturally became a light sleeper. It took me eleven months after my father's passing, before I slept through an entire night. I found myself tossing and turning, stuck in the habit of being concerned about him nocturnally.

Everyone needs sleep, and dealing with the additional stress of being a caregiver, the human body will require even more. It is a well-known fact that sleep is essential to maintaining good health. You can only skimp on sleep for a short period of time before major compilations start setting in. Going without enough rest for extended lengths of time will cause a variety of drastic conditions to develop, such as weight gain, irritability, depression and other mental and physical disorders.

When your patient's symptoms begin to move forward, sleep deprivation will become a more frequent problem. Fatigue will creep up to the point where you can't even see straight. Accompanying headaches and body pains could last for days.

There were times when I would call my sister so she could come sit with our father so I could just sleep; and the fact I knew I didn't have to worry about him would let me get some of the soundest sleep I'd had in weeks.

When you're exhausted, mistakes are easily made and being a caregiver, you could commit an error that could be disastrous!

You must learn to ask for help. You need someone who can pitch in. If you have a nearby relative, don't

take "no" for an answer. You can't go without sleeping. Everything will certainly fall apart and then there
will be two people in dire need of help.

The main point here is that you're indispensable.
If you stall out, there will be one heck of a traffic jam.
Keep your oil changed and don't miss those scheduled
tune-ups, otherwise the next sound you hear may be
the mixture of metal and hydraulics as you're being
towed away.

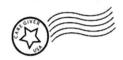

Dear Caregiver,

Author and campaigner for the blind, Helen Adams Keller wrote: "Your success and happiness lies in you. Resolve to keep happy, and your joy and you shall form an invincible host against difficulties."

GJL

Coping with Caregiver Guilt

Guilt is an overpowering and complicated emotion but appears to have a purpose in the life of human beings. Upon realizing that we've done something wrong, by all means, we should experience a touch of shame.

If you are a caregiver, there will be times when waves of guilt will wash right over you. There doesn't have to be any wrongdoing involved. The simple reason is that you care so deeply that you never feel adequate enough to perform this role.

For example, you may finally get a chance to do something for yourself. Let's say you go out to get an overdue haircut. The whole time you're sitting in the salon chair, you can't stop thinking about something bad happening while you are away. You rush straight home, instead of taking advantage of the rare and well-deserved respite break. Even when you find, to your relief, that all is well, you still experience that guilt monster.

Here's another scenario: Your mother calls you first thing in the morning. She just wants to talk with you because the sound of your voice is comforting to her, but because she suffers from dementia, she forgets she called you three times already and has been calling every ten minutes! By the sixth phone call (and seeing it's her phone number once again on the caller ID screen) you elect not to answer. Within minutes, guilt starts swirling around inside you. "What if something has really happened to her?" Next thing you know you're breaking speed limits, driving to her house to make sure everything is okay!

Then there's always that "little white lie." You may be visiting your loved one at his or her adult living facility or the hospital. You need to be at work in a couple of hours yet, but you like to have at least one hour to yourself before you begin your shift. Suddenly you find yourself saying, "My boss asked if I could come in early today so I'm going to have to leave now." Meanwhile, throughout your whole work shift, you once again feel guilt doing somersaults in your stomach.

There's not a caregiver out there that doesn't question whether or not the job he or she is doing is good enough. Even after your loved one has passed away you will go through a stage of beating yourself up, wondering whether or not there was something more you could have done.

The strong emotion of guilt that caregivers endure is just part of human nature. Go to a caregiver support group and ask all those surrounding you. They will tell you that they too are experiencing or have experienced the exact same feelings. All caregivers face the same unattainable goal of sparing their loved ones the pain that comes with any disease. Everyone's desire is to provide a compassionate passing.

Deep inside, we all believe that we, as caregivers, are to some degree responsible for what happens to our stricken loved ones in the end. Sadly, some endings can be downright cruel, not only to the one afflicted with the disease but also to the ones that have to witness the perishing.

Caregivers get hit with a double whammy. While trying to wade through all the sadness and grief, they get swept away by a pronounced tide of guilt. But take heart; this guilt trip will slowly start to fade, finally leaving you with just the normal amount of grief, which is difficult enough.

With the passing of your loved one, life has just spun around 180 degrees. Everything you have trained yourself to do has come to a complete halt. That grueling fast-paced lifestyle you were living has just stopped itself on a dime. It's almost as if you have to learn to breathe all over again.

Try not to berate yourself about areas in which you think you may have failed. Instead, focus on all the positive things you accomplished along the way. Think of the enhanced quality of life you singlehandedly brought to your loved one. Remember, you will remain in his or her heart forever.

Unfortunately, guilt is a normal emotion in life. These bouts of guilt you feel only prove what a caring individual you truly are.

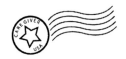

Dear Caregiver,

Louis L'Amour once said: "There will come a time when you believe everything is finished; that will be the beginning."

I believe that when this campaign is over, you will find this to be so true.

GJL

Backup

(Designing a Backup Plan)

Accidents happen. This well-known fact makes it imperative for the caregiver to devise a backup plan. This plan must be designed to have another person available who can take over responsibilities in case of emergencies.

Let's say you trip over something and sprain or break your ankle. While you're sitting with your foot elevated, the Alzheimer's patient you're caring for will constantly ask, "What happened to your foot?" You know how tiring it is to be asked over and over about your injuries. Well, now you will be asked twenty to thirty times a day and that's probably an extremely low estimate.

So now you'll be hobbling around, trying to care for the both of you. This is not a good scenario—trust me, I've been there.

It is the primary caregiver's responsibility to make sure there's someone always ready, willing and trained to step in when there's an emergency. I'm not just talking about broken bones here; there are doctors' appointments, medications, financial matters, etc. The list is long and you know it. What happens if you die? Make certain ahead of time that the fate of your loved one will be placed in the right hands. If you have power of attorney, papers need to be drawn up to have someone responsible enough to take charge should you not be there. Do you really want the court to decide? No? I didn't think so. Unfortunately, if this actually happens, you won't be here. Decisions must be made now! Meet with your attorney and have the appropriate papers drawn up. Explain the entire situation and that someone must be able to legally make the proper decisions in your absence. Since the one you're caring for is unable to handle his or her own affairs, you must get busy immediately on this master plan.

You, as the caregiver, are of the utmost importance in the life of your loved one. Meet with your family members or friends and put a backup plan together. You never know when something could happen.

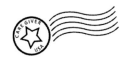

Dear Caregiver,

Poet Haniel Long wrote:"So much of what is best in us is bound up in our love of family that it remains the measure of our stability because it measures our sense of loyalty. All other pacts of love or fear derive from it and are modeled upon it."

The fact that your loved one has you standing by their side has given them an encouraging edge to make it more peaceful through this campaign.

GJL

A Tough Kind of Love

(Caregiving Hardships and Removing Driving Privileges)

Personally watching a loved one dissolve in front of your eyes is one of the hardest undertakings a caregiver must endure.

Abiding at my father's side for nearly a decade, observing the disheartening deterioration caused by Alzheimer's, I can honestly say that I knew my father better than he knew himself.

Early on, convincing Dad to get a medical opinion about his memory loss was difficult, to say the least. Thus began my role as his primary caregiver. Obtaining a diagnosis is really the first step of caring for a loved one with Alzheimer's. No one wants to hear they have acquired a fatal mind-robbing disease—especially from a family member. Even coming from a doctor, such a diagnosis strikes like lightning. Of course, my dad claimed the doctor was out of his cotton-pickin' mind. "Who cares if I can't find my pencil?" I wouldn't want to count the times I heard that one. But having a diagnosis will benefit you and your loved one in several ways.

Putting a halt the driving privileges of those suffering from Alzheimer's is inevitable. It is also one of the most difficult tasks a caregiver or a family member will ever face. Driving a car is one of the last stands of independence a person will fight to retain. Once traveling to and from is no longer possible, dependence upon others becomes a necessity.

While still in the early stage of Alzheimer's, the operating of a motor vehicle may still be an option, but this time period doesn't last long. Family members need to watch for significant signs, alerting them to when it is time to step in. Some common indications can be as the following: getting lost in familiar areas, driving too fast or too slow, ignoring traffic signs and becoming easily upset or angry. One thing is for sure, we don't need anymore road rage.

When the day comes that you've decided enough is enough, you must be firm and resolute. The subject cannot be open to discussion. "Well, you seem fairly clear-headed today. I guess you'll be okay." No, it doesn't work that way. They could be fine pulling out of the driveway and then two miles down the road become drenched in confusion, unable to find their way home.

My father's last driving experience was an outing to the post office. He drove himself there to mail out his monthly bills and pick up any mail deposited in our post office box. He got himself halfway home, then turned around to mail the bills he already sent. Unable to find the already mailed envelopes, he worked himself into a fluster. He started driving home and spun the car around once again. He finally arrived home three and a half hours later as white as a ghost. I made sure that was the last time he ever drove a car. If I knew then the information I'm about to tell you now, I could have made the undertaking of this nondriving campaign much less tormenting. I simply informed my dad that his doctor had called the Motor Vehicle Department (MVD) and had his license revoked. This brought on months of four letter words and proclamations that the state department must be brainless for listening to his doctor (who he swore he'd never see again).

Now I've discovered that most MVDs have a link on their Website that directs you to a document called "Medical Reporting Form" which you can fill out anonymously.

Next, the person in question will receive an appointment in the mail to take an on road driving test (ORDT) which they must pass to maintain their driving privileges. Recent studies report that patients with mild Alzheimer's disease who failed the ORDT all consider themselves to be safe drivers.

I will warn you right now that once you embark on this covert operation, everything changes. Suddenly loved ones will have 101 places to go every day. Sadly, this is also a stage where massive depression starts seeping in. But you can no longer let them behind the wheel where they could possibly hurt either themselves or others.

It will take awhile, but eventually they will accept being chauffeured around. And they will also become more and more comfortable staying in the safety of their own home.

Make no mistake, this is hard. You'll need help. Take all you can get. You will go through stages when you feel strong, and you are! It requires a special individual to be caregiver to memory-impaired persons. But anticipate that you will get worn down. That burnout stage does absolutely nothing but cause harm for everybody. So put your pride aside and let others help. This is a job that can't be done alone. I knew when that level of feebleness was about to drag me into the dirt and I was guilty as sin of ignoring any forewarning signs. I should have practiced what I preach, especially on this subject.

One problem with the burnout stage is that you'll never really get a chance to recuperate. What's even worse is when you get sick with such illnesses as the flu, cold, headache or a migraine. When you're feeling ill, it's hard not to lose your patience.

This is where you must have an alternative plan. You will need a medical diagnosis in order to receive any kind of home care. This includes Hospice and any others down the road. Also have a person or persons you can call on to cover for you in case of emergencies. When you find these extraordinary persons, let them slowly become part of the routine lifestyle you have worked to establish. This way they will get used to the way the household is run and patients won't be pushed into an anxiety attack when left with a stranger; plan ahead before disaster strikes.

People with Alzheimer's will go through a period when the frustration just crushes them. This is an unavoidable event in the evolution of a mind that is stricken with Alzheimer's, but trust me, it will ease up, hopefully for a good long run.

Hang tough. It's important that loved ones know that they can always count on their caregiver. As hard as it becomes, you will have to bear with them.

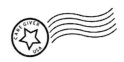

Dear Caregiver,

Peter Ustinov came up with a statement that really hit home: "Parents are the bones on which children sharpen their teeth."

If you're caring for an ill parent, it's more than likely you inherited that good heart of yours from them.

GJL

Essence

(Patients' Personalities and Unpredictable Behavior)

The dread of failure is every caregiver's nightmare. Try to relax and observe your loved one closely. Learn as much as possible day-to-day. Don't be so hard on yourself. Remember that every Alzheimer's patient responds differently in most instances.

The original personality will never totally vanish. If your father or mother were jokesters, you better stay on your toes! They might be planning their next caper after many years into this disease. Enjoy these moments and remind yourself hour by hour that your patient has no concept of time.

Again, learn from these people. One of the reasons why I get so aggravated with the medical profession is that the vast majority of doctors and nurses refuse to listen to the caregivers or patients. You are the foreman. Obviously there are many reasons that you have to accompany them to that doctor's appointment. Memory-impaired patients cannot answer for themselves. You might be the only one around who recognizes when they're just playing tomfoolery.

Many will categorize a person with Alzheimer's as mentally encumbered. Well, my father struggled with the disease for over ten years and always maintained a sense of humor, regardless of all the depression that culprit of a disease rained down upon him. Except for an earlier stage, when the frustration became overwhelming, his personality always remained his own.

One of the most challenging symptoms of Alzheimer's is the constant change of behavior. This characteristic can often be the deciding factor in a family's decision to place their loved one in a residential care facility.

Behavioral and psychiatric symptoms of Alzheimer's patients can include a large group of side effects, such as aggression, agitation, confusion, suspicion, hallucinations and that's just to name a few.

The sudden change in a patient's demeanor can appear suddenly without any prewarning or logical reason. A large percentage seems to develop from frustrations, growing anxiety and fear that can cause your loved one to act out in anger or burst out sobbing in tears.

Trying to predict these mood swings is a difficult thing to master. Each situation is unique. One woman told me that the worst part of her day was usually the first part of the morning, when caring for her Alzheimer's-stricken husband. Myself, I had more hardships with my father during the evenings when he would experience Sundowner's, otherwise known as "Sundown Syndrome."

There are an abundance of theories about what sets off these shifting behaviors. Among them can even be physical discomfort or poor environmental conditions. Whatever the cause, once again I believe that keeping to a daily routine is the best preventive measure. Limit as many distractions as possible and speak slowly in a soft, calming tone. If they begin to become agitated, try shifting their focus to a fresh and relaxing activity, such as listening to quiet music, taking a walk together, watching the sunset, etc.

If combativeness is involved, take a step back and draw in a couple of deep breaths. This will help you release any adrenalin building in your system so you may remain calm. If both of you become worked up, this is a battle no one will ever win.

Once you have yourself in the right state of mind, provide reassurance that they are safe. Promise that you will stay by their side until everything is better and make sure the environment is comfortable.

Take away any unnecessary chatter; ask whoever is in the room to leave until the situation is resolved.

If these plights start becoming more frequent, talk to a physician. There are several medications which help control anxiety. This worked well for my dad.

Learn to be aware of the warning signs. Watch for restlessness, fidgeting or pacing. This may be a good time to ask if they would enjoy going for a walk. Search for any safe outlet that will release the escalating energy. Things like asking if they would like to help you with the dishes will keep their hands and minds occupied and possibly assist you in avoiding any emotional explosions.

Remember . . . never, ever argue with them. It is not only pointless but will only cause to provoke your loved one further.

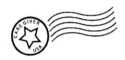

Dear Caregiver,

One of the many things I've learned through my caregiving journey is that when patients have hallucinations or become delusional—don't try to talk them out of whatever they think they're seeing. It's as real to them as the ground you're standing on.

GJL

Why Don't You See Them?

(Hallucinations and Delusions)

"They're breaking into the building next door! All the tools behind the building are being stolen!" Over and over Dad kept repeating this throughout an afternoon. I walked him over there four or five times in hopes that it would settle him down.

This is only one of the cruel effects of Alzheimer's and was one of the hardest for me to bear. He had been suffering from this pillaging disease for practically a decade, and what I've just described is one of its most heartrending facets.

Hallucinations and delusions are two of the most strenuous side effects for a caregiver to contend with. You will really need to pull out all your endurance in order to avoid losing your patience. Exhibiting signs of frustration will make matters worse.

Years ago, on a Memorial Day weekend, Dad took a gander out the kitchen window and asked, "What are those twenty-five people doing having dinner in our backyard?" Now, as you know by now, I would never have even considered inviting that many guests. I always persisted in preserving him in a simple routine lifestyle, keeping all confusion at a minimum. Truly, I believe that this is your most important asset in assisting a patient with Alzheimer's. Keep it simple.

If it happens that your patient truly believes he or she is witnessing something, don't turn it into a debate. *Period!* Instead, be affirming with, "I just went out and checked. They must have just left." You might have to take a walk outside and circle the house. At this point, you probably need some fresh air and some good ol' dirt kicking. Whatever you do, don't get into an argument. It will only twist things further and you both will likely be headed for hours of extended madness.

I confess that this was one of the most difficult situations I had to deal with as caregiver. There were many times it became necessary to call my beloved sister for backup because I couldn't handle Dad's delusions one more minute. Like a "horse rode too hard and put up wet," I needed open pasture and Sis came to the rescue. Get the point? Alzheimer's patients can use you up. I considered going for a long drive, but while my sister sat with him, I decided just to sleep. I was simply too mentally and physically exhausted to go anywhere.

It's amazing how the untrue will remain in patients' minds sometimes for days, but then in a moment, something that just happened two minutes ago no longer exists.

What they believe they're seeing, smelling or even tasting is as real to them as the love you possess that keeps you going.

Dear Caregiver,

David Letterman, host of "The Late Show" said something that really amused me: "Be suspicious of any doctor who tries to take your temperature with his finger."

GJL

Alzheimer's Doctors

(Choosing or Switching Physicians and Memory Tests)

"I'm not receiving enough help from our doctor," is perhaps the most common complaint I hear from Alzheimer's caregivers. I certainly understand their concern. I ended up switching doctors myself. It's my opinion that since there is no cure, some physicians become stagnant and just are not aggressive enough, not realizing there are two people in need of care—the patient and the caregiver.

You should know it's difficult switching to a new doctor. There's a feeling of security in staying with the same one for a lengthy period of time. Then there is also a concern about hurting the doctor's feelings after building a doctor—patient relationship.

If it should become necessary to find a new physician, be sure that expectations can be reasonably met.

Often, caregivers become overtired and worn down, so be sure to make this decision with careful thought when well rested.

Be aware that changing physicians will be time consuming and may incur additional cost such as copying and transferring medical files along with requiring new lab tests.

Your first question should be, "What type of doctor treats Alzheimer's patients?" A primary care physician should be able to handle all your routine needs. However, should you need a specialist for other medical concerns, neurologists, geriatric psychiatrists and geriatricians all receive training in evaluation and treatment of memory disorders.

My advice to you is to see if you can iron things out with your doctor first. Remember that any type of change is difficult for an Alzheimer's patient. Ask for a moment alone with your physician to explain how you feel and what changes need to be made to best care for your patient. If your doctor is not willing to listen and consider your concerns, you have your answer. Make a change.

The health-care community appears to have become sluggish in their ability to recognize mild memory impairment or early stage Alzheimer's. This tells me that we still have a long way to go in educating both the public and private sector regarding this life-destroying disease.

Quite frequently, the first reaction when a loved one seems to start making simple mistakes is just to pardon it off as, "Well, he or she is starting to get up there in age." But continue to pursue answers since early detection of Alzheimer's or dementia is essential in the administration of medications and also the making of a significant game plan.

There appears to be one trait resulting from Alzheimer's. It seems to appear in both the victims and most everyone who is close to them, and that trait is denial.

When my father first started showing signs of dementia, I had it stuck in my head that he may be suffering from ministrokes, also known as transient ischemic attack (TIA). When he was diagnosed with Alzheimer's, it just straight-out hurt.

There are many physicians who are also in denial or might actually feel that when patients are so far into their senior years, there is no reason for them to receive the same aggressive treatments as the young. Instead, in today's world, they should assiduously be taught to say, "Because of their age they should have a memory test administered."

The United States Prevention Task Force, formed of an independent panel of experts in primary care and preventive medicine, now recommends that physicians assess all patients for dementia when there is a question of cognition impairment.

Currently, the most commonly used test is the minimental state exam (MMSE). During the beginning process of this test, there are three different objects mentioned. Next, the patient may be asked to spell a word backward or asked to describe something in particular. Finally, the doctor ends the test by asking, "What were the first three objects mentioned?"

There is also a test being performed called "test your memory" (TYM) which is appearing to be more accurate. It requires patients to complete ten simple tasks; things like completing a simple math equation or explaining what two certain objects have in common. For example, can you give me four proper first names beginning with the letter "C" and of course, the ol' draw a face of a clock with the hands pointing to a certain time assigned by the doctor.

According to the experts, this test has identified close to 90 percent of patients which were surmised of having Alzheimer's. Meanwhile, the MMSE test showed only half that amount. Researchers are currently doing further tests to validate these results.

Alzheimer's makes up about 65 percent of all dementia-related conditions. It is by far the more common dementia disease. These days this also is a cause for mistaken diagnosis. Sadly, many diseases that are reversible, unlike Alzheimer's, may be pushed aside.

Here is a list of some of the diseases that are commonly misdiagnosed as Alzheimer's: Lewy body dementia, Parkinson's disease, Huntington's disease, Creutzfeldt-Jakob disease, normal pressure hydrocephalus, Pick's disease, multi-infarct dementia, also known as vascular dementia and depression.

Currently, doctors are taught in medical school to rule out all the reversible causes first.

If there was one thing I received from all my years of caregiving, it was a first-class education in patience. Don't jump to the wrong conclusion. Wait for all the test results to be in and hopefully the problem will be reversible, unlike the fatal disease of Alzheimer's.

Remember, second opinions are of great value in the determination of causes of dementia of any kind. And checking twice may reveal the good news that it's reversible.

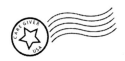

Dear Caregiver,

American humorist Franklin P. Jones said: "Anybody who thinks talk is cheap should get some legal advice."

The price you pay for legal advice could be only a fraction of what you might be paying without it.

GJL

Sign Here, Please

(Power of Attorney and Health-care Surrogate)

Loved ones who have been diagnosed with Alzheimer's require more than being attended to for mental and physical ailments. Honest, meticulous care for their financial matters must be addressed as well from the very day they are diagnosed.

At the first opportunity, a financial plan should be organized for their future. The whimsical declaration of "we've got plenty of time" will sneak up and bite you in the behind. The truth is that there is no time! A caregiver's schedule can become so hectic that they barely have time to remember to breathe.

One of the first signs of my father's memory loss was noticing that his bills were being paid late or not at all. This was so out of character for him. I started writing out his checks, then having him sign them. This turned into a two-hour session, I began to dread. He would tortuously question me over and over whether a certain paid bill had not already been paid earlier.

An attorney needs to be contacted. Ascertain whether he or she has expertise in public benefit. Due to the memory impairment of Alzheimer's, appropriate papers need to be drawn up without delay. Remember, as time elapses, chances increase for a claim to arise that the patient wasn't competent at the time of executing the protective legal documents.

Someone who is completely trustworthy needs to be designated Durable Power of Attorney, and whomever acquires this position must fall into a strict habit of signing his or her name ending with P.O.A. every single time a document is signed for the patient. Also, it must be realized that the power of attorney will cease to exist the minute the patient passes away. Anything signed incorrectly could come back hauntingly.

Most medical and financial institutions have absolutely no heart. They'll start calling mere days after the passing of your loved one. You can ease most future burdens yourself by lawfully adding those three little letters to your signature: P.O.A.

Other institutions I discovered to often have ruthless, frigid hearts are banks and investment groups. Most of them will be reluctant or even unwilling to accept your Durable Power of Attorney. It might be in your benefit to set up a joint checking account as soon as possible so to insure bills can be paid in a timely fashion. Make sure the bank account reads "*or*" not "*and.*" This will keep the account active after your loved ones' passing.

Every competent adult has the fundamental right to make self-determined decisions pertaining to his or her own health. This is why having a living will in place ahead of time is essential.

A living will is a written document concerning one's wishes regarding medical treatment in the event he or she cannot make these decisions for themselves. Contained in this legal paper will be the name of a legally appointed health-care surrogate. It will become his or her job to determine necessary care in case the wind has been knocked out of the named person's sails due to illness, accidents, etc.

Of course, every family is different. One may have an older son who is trustworthy in the handling of finances when at the same time a younger daughter is the one gifted in making medical decisions. This is where choosing a health-care surrogate comes in.

Designation of a health-care surrogate should be made through a written document and be signed in the presence of two witnesses, one of whom is neither a spouse nor blood relative. The person assigned as the surrogate cannot be a witness at all.

Always keep the original document in your personal files where it is accessible to others if needed. Have all physicians' concerned place a copy in the named person's medical records and, if hospitalized, bring a copy with you each and every time he or she is admitted. Your assigned surrogate also needs to maintain a copy in his or her file and one might also consider leaving a copy with a spiritual advisor.

Another precaution is to name an alternate surrogate for backup in case the primary surrogate is unavailable or unable to serve.

If you have an existing living will or advance care plan and you decide to make a change, destroy all copies. In the event you have no plan put together and you are found lacking mental competence, it will be up to your doctor to appoint a surrogate. There is a set standard by which that person is selected. The first on the list is your spouse. Next in line would be one of your adult children, thirdly a parent, and then an adult grandchild or possibly even a close friend.

You might wonder how the doctor decides when a patient is unable to make his or her own medical decisions. There are two methods a physician, psychologist or advance nurse practitioner utilizes in making this determination; one has been the evaluation of a person's ability to appreciate the nature and implications of a health-care decision and the other is the person's ability or inability to communicate personal choice in an unambiguous manner.

For example, I had to decide whether to prolong my father's suffering and have a feeding tube inserted into his stomach. I decided based on what I knew his wishes would be that he had suffered long enough.

Personally, I believe the best thing to do is to assign a Medical Power of Attorney. This way you can specify in writing what health-care decisions can or cannot be made.

There is a lot of anguish and potential guilt for the persons designated and whether they made the right choices. This is why it is so important for you, the potential patient, to sit down with the person you have chosen (and other family members) and clarify exactly what your wishes are.

Make sure that your prolonging or end-of-life desires will be correctly carried out; make a living will and choose a health-care surrogate before it is too late to do so.

Call a family meeting ASAP. It might take several gatherings before anything gets accomplished but don't give up. I can't stress how important it is to get things in order immediately.

Dear Caregiver,

American psychoanalyst and author Theodore Isaac Rubin said:"Kindness is more important than wisdom, and the recognition of this is the beginning of wisdom."

In other words, don't worry about the mistakes that are going to be made; it's more important that you learn from them.

GJL

A Caregiver's Promise

(Patient Confidentiality)

When caring for an Alzheimer's patient, you may hear them utter things that are so far off the wall there's no making heads or tails of what they're talking about. But keep in mind, if you really listen to this chatter, you might come across some statements said that should never be repeated to anyone.

"Patient confidentiality" is a trust and bond that should be taken seriously by everyone who works in the health-care profession. This rule should even apply to the person doing the much needed job of housekeeping.

Privacy is a public right and we, as a society, have an ethical obligation to protect the memory impaired. Patients could be having what seems like a normal conversation with just anyone when suddenly they become paranoid that everyone is against them, talking about them behind their backs and stealing all their belongings. Next they will demand that you go out to the backyard and start digging up coffee cans full of money they buried behind the big oak tree. Chances are that the money was already dug up some twenty years ago, if it ever existed at all!

There can always be an exception to the rule. In a situation like this, the patient's legal guardian or their power of attorney should be informed. But remember, it may not just have to do with money. I have heard several stories of patients burying their guns in the backyard. Obviously, this information needs to be investigated immediately.

Another frequent problem when dealing with Alzheimer's patients is that they rarely give the same answer to a question twice. So when they claim they're having chest pains or some other type of body aches, they should be taken seriously the first time and their physician be immediately notified. Don't ignore other complaints but use discretion in discerning the severity.

And still another significant concern is "identity theft." Just in the United States alone, an estimated 13.3 people have their identity stolen every minute. It's a part of the caregiver's job to make sure that patients aren't being forgetful or foolishly mishandling their wallet or purse. The responsibility of keeping them safe involves more than just their physical well-being.

Even when caregivers are out enjoying what little social life they have, they must remain on their toes and not spill out any personal information that could cause the patient harm. There's always someone out there waiting to prey on the people who are most vulnerable. There's an old saying "between you and me and the lamppost." Well, leave the lamppost and the other person out of this. If unwarranted questions are asked about your loved one, simply answer, "It would be inappropriate for me to answer that."

Today's technology lends itself to the thievery of personal information. If faxing important documents, be sure to remove the original papers from the machine. In addition, sensitive e-mails should always be deleted.

I personally know how stressful and demanding the job of being a caregiver is, and I hate to add more worries on top of the ones you already have. But these people are depending on you and if that bond of trust becomes compromised, they may start holding back vital information like severe symptoms they're experiencing.

A true caregiver-patient relationship must be built on honest-to-goodness trust. Stay faithful to your loved one. Loyalty is everything to them.

Dear Caregiver,

Comedienne Ellen DeGeneres amusingly quipped: "My grandmother started walking five miles a day when she was sixty. She's ninety-three today and we don't know where the hell she is." This definitely reminded me of Alzheimer's patients' wandering.

GJL

The Wanderer

(Wandering)

One morning at 2:35 a.m., I was awakened to the familiar clanking sound of my father's walker. Lying still, I listened closely to assure myself that I actually heard Dad moving around. Suddenly, the distinctive sound of the backdoor opening brought me instantly to my feet. "Where are we going?" I asked as if we were a team. "I've got to take a leak," was his retort.

Dad's confusion, brought on by Alzheimer's, had him believing he was still in his childhood home where the only plumbing was the outhouse in the backyard. This was an extremely dangerous situation. Just the darkness alone would have magnified his confusion to the point where he might not have found his way back to the house. He might have fallen, lying there for hours. Morning would dawn and he would have been nowhere to be found.

I was fortunate that my father wasn't very mobile; he needed a walking device which, thankfully, rattled louder than a provoked rattlesnake. Believe me, I went through my share of warning devices that alerted me when he was on the move.

First was a baby monitor hidden in his bedroom closet. I was quite impressed with the clarity of how well it picked up every little sound. It even resounded the toilet flushing, but after lying awake night after night listening to him snore, I moved on to another device which proved to be less than a stroke of genius: stuffed parrots with motion detectors built inside that squawked loud enough to wake the dead when anyone passed by. Positioned at the front and backdoor, they worked extremely well except for the fact that they almost gave everybody heart attacks. I finally moved on to placing dead bolts at the top of the doorframes. The only problem I had with this was that he occasionally locked me out of the house.

Find out what works best for your situation. There are many variables when dealing with memory-impaired patients. Remember, every Alzheimer's patient responds differently.

Remember, as the disease advances communication skills quickly evaporate. Be creative; try placing signs throughout the house indicating which way to turn to go to which room. I positioned a sign on the bathroom door with great success. You can write it out or just place a picture of a toilet on it. Many times when you find them roaming about, it's only because they couldn't remember what they originally started out to do. Random background noise could also be a contributing factor. For instance, the sound of someone knocking on a television program might send them to the front door; one more step, and they're outside wandering away.

You could have them wear an ID bracelet. Many organizations have a "safe return program" where you can have one made. If they're still carrying a wallet, make sure that it contains a list of contact numbers and addresses.

There are Websites designed for caregiver's and family members alike to file vital information that would be needed in case a loved one wanders from home; this file contains current photos, addresses, phone numbers and all crucial background information needed for police departments and possibly search and rescue teams. This data can be downloaded in a minute's time.

But it is essential for caregivers to update their data approximately every six months. There's no doubt that many Alzheimer's patients get shuffled around. For instance, I know of a family in which the daughter tried taking care of an afflicted parent but only to find out, months later, she just couldn't handle it. Soon the patient ended up at another sibling's home, and then an adult facility. You can almost count on most of the paperwork and vital information being lost in the shuffle.

Updating photos are also important. Just from the vast weight loss during my father's last year, many of his past acquaintances would never have recognized him.

Obviously, we need to use all of the new technology available to us, such as locator bands which produce a miniaturized single-purpose cell phone designed to be worn like a wristwatch. Not to be mistaken for Dick Tracy's two-way radio watch, this device, only upon activation, dials 911 and reports its location. It works solely upon existing emergency 911 systems and needs to be charged approximately two hours every week.

I've written several times about how every patient responds differently. In my father's situation, he wasn't very mobile. He needed a walker to assist him which made his wandering a limited problem only throughout his earlier years of the disease, not that he wouldn't have wandered later on if he could.

Accidents can happen in microseconds. One foot over the threshold and there is no telling what could happen next.

Being lost will compound their confusion and they might become belligerent or verbally abusive. Strangers just trying to help them might be in for a handful.

I have a close friend whose father suffered from the same dreadful disease. Once she had the police department along with their recovery dogs searching for her dad for almost a full day. They finally discovered him sitting alone in someone's living room chair, wearing his new host's pink fluffy slippers. He was in a similar-looking apartment in the same complex, watching television and eating ice cream. No harm came to him, but this was a somewhat comical ending to what could have been a potentially tragic chain of events.

Temperature extremes and inclement weather should be another major concern for any caregiver who is watching over an elderly person. The body's ability to produce its own heat declines with age. In addition, those suffering from Alzheimer's or other forms of dementia bring on additional worries during a cold spell.

You'd think that you wouldn't have to worry about loved ones venturing outside into freezing temperatures. After all, who would want to go face the elements and be anesthetized by the blistering cold? But the fact remains that any change in climate will cause an interruption in their daily routine, bringing on heavier bouts of confusion. Suddenly, you may find them moving from room to room searching for additional warmth. Be aware that hypothermia is a danger lurking around many corners.

Hypothermia comes from the lowering of the body temperature to ninety-five degrees Fahrenheit or below. I know that my father's body temperature would normally stay around ninety-seven degrees Fahrenheit, which put him almost halfway to being at risk.

Even in moderately cool temperatures, around forty-five degrees Fahrenheit hypothermia can occur. All it takes is a person becoming chilled from being caught in the rain or even soaked from their own sweat.

Hypothermia is a medical emergency that requires immediate attention. Some indications will be as follows: decreased heart and respiratory rates, slow reflexes, shivering and additional confusion. It may also cause the victim to suffer from oxygen deprivation, causing an inability for them to comprehend that they are in dire need of help which would likely prevent them from seeking shelter. They may likewise lose the ability to communicate how they actually feel.

If you're not living with the ones you're caring for 24/7, explain to their neighbors what the situation is and ask them to check on them and call you immediately if they see them wandering away from home.

Even if they live in a care facility, the concern about them wandering doesn't go away. Every year, there are many cases of patients dying after roaming away from adult living centers. The official medical term for this is "elopement." Always look into each living establishment's ability to cope with this before deciding to place your loved one there. Keep in mind that even if he or she never had a history of wandering, this doesn't mean it's not going to happen in the near future. An interesting diversion can be to hide a favorite "going out hat" or purse, suppressing the desire to leave.

Just try to make sure patients reside in comfortable surroundings. You don't want them to become cold in the middle of the night, causing them to begin to roam around, possibly getting into trouble.

The dangers involved when a wandering memory-impaired patient is unsupervised are endless.

Comfort Prayers

Beyond our grief and unknown fears

above anxiety and tears,

there's something bigger than it all

someone greater answers our call.

Our grace is strengthened and renewed

when we are filled with gratitude.

Something within, deep inside

lets us know good things abide.

Ester Marie Latz

Motor Skills

(Loss of Physical and Mental Abilities)

All throughout the last decade of my father's life, I watched him deteriorate from Alzheimer's. Not only did I witness his memory disintegrate to the point where he no longer recognized his own family but, sadly, I observed his motor skills reluctantly evaporate.

I began to notice the development of a shuffle in his walk and I tried convincing myself that it was because he was in his eighties, surmising it was only natural for him to lose a step or two. Age wasn't the problem. The fact was that the Alzheimer's was causing his equilibrium to dissipate daily. Also he had become nervous, always hesitating before taking his next step.

His hands began to shake to the point where he could barely get a spoon to his mouth. He also suffered from involuntary muscle movements and slow reflexes. The regression of his motor skills was caused directly by the disease itself.

So much more is affected from this illness other than just being memory impaired. Dementia is only one of the symptoms of this heartless disease. The list is horrendously long and sad.

People with this malady will often lose muscle mass. According to a report from the *Journal of the American Medical Association* (JAMA), "The weight loss of a person's muscle, bone and internal organs—rather than only body fat—was linked to an increased likelihood of Alzheimer's disease."

An in-depth study was made of men and women who were afflicted with the disease and also those who were not. The percentage of total body fat between the two groups was about the same.

But the study suggests that the brains of those afflicted with the disease disrupted the nervous system's ability to regulate energy throughout the body. I'm sure that parts of these results are due to the patient becoming less and less active.

Please remember, as our loved ones' skills start slipping away, they are still the same person who we learned to love and admire. They are just going to need more and more assistance. This obviously means that the need to rely on you, the caregiver, will likely become overwhelming. But this is what makes a caregiver such a special person.

Here are a few suggestions which may help tremendously when their motor skills start slipping away:

- Eliminate silverware by serving finger foods
- Exchange buttons for Velcro
- Provide sweat pants (no zippers)

Try to assist your loved one to maintain as much independence for as long as possible. If he or she can still perform a certain task, allow for it. Preserving self-respect will help a long way through this infuriating ordeal.

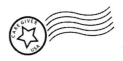

Dear Caregiver,

Titus Maccius Plautus, a Roman playwright said: "Nothing but heaven itself is better than a friend who is really a friend."

Being caregiver is not just the act of caring for someone, it's also the act of true friendship.

GJL

Body Language

(Communication Skills,
The Five W's and Speech Therapy)

Once afflicted with Alzheimer's, a loved one will start losing their communication skills. Unfortunately, it's inevitable. As a caregiver, you need to adjust your speaking techniques throughout the different stages of the disease, adapting to changes as they occur.

Learn to face the patients directly, talking to them as if they're reading your lips. I'll be the first to admit I was guilty of saying something to my dad as I was walking into another room, only to have to return and speak in a more direct manner, making sure he clearly understood me.

Be patient with them and yourself. This matter gets very frustrating and tiresome. Learn to stay away from subjects that might upset them. I won't make a list of subjects to avoid as this is unique to each individual.

You'll know which ones they are. If you don't, you'll quickly figure them out by the other responses you get as time goes by.

In some of the more orthodox crime detective practices of solving mysteries, trained investigators are taught to always concentrate on asking the five W's: who, what, when, where and why. As a caregiver, you will soon discover that your daily routine involves the perpetual task of solving many mysteries. But, on the other hand, these are also five words you will want to refrain from using at certain times.

Common sense should be telling you when to back away from any questions which are incorporated with the five W's.

- *Who* are you upset with?
- *What* do you think you're doing?
- *When* are you going to wash up?
- *Where* do you think you're going?
- *Why* are you crying?

There are many other letters in the alphabet besides W's to worry about. The point being, when you see that they are already having difficulties, don't begin making inquiries that you know they probably won't be able to answer, likely causing further turmoil. Just use the five W's as a rule of thumb to hold in abeyance in the back of your mind.

The short-term memory will gradually dissipate from the mind of Alzheimer's patients. Whatever happened just a few minutes ago never occurred in the mind of these victims. However, the long-term memory survives until the latter stage of the disease.

My father's memories of his many siblings and buddies from the past always seemed to remain fresh. This has me believing that if old friends are still available, any social interaction with them, even if it's just a weekly phone conversation, could be very therapeutic, possibly helping to keep your loved ones' long-term memory and communication skills viable longer.

Caregivers should make it their goal to maintain patients' verbal abilities extending as far into the disease as feasible. Once they stop speaking, everything else begins accelerating downhill from that point.

Do what you can to encourage quiet social visits or phone conversations with figures from the past. They may hang up the receiver, instantly forgetting whom they just talked with, but the mental exercise of that conversation just might keep their long-term gears turning. You'll want to stay within earshot of the confabulation just in case they begin to become flustered.

A fellow caregiver explained to me that her mother is constantly asking if she can move back to her hometown. Her mom believes that everything would go back to the way things were forty some years ago and she would be living the same lifestyle of her younger days. Now we all know this isn't possible, but what would be the harm in letting her exchange fifteen minutes of friendly chitchat, reminiscing with an old sidekick from the days she can still remember.

At one point during my dad's illness, I began noticing randomly dialed numbers showing up on my phone bill. It's probably a good idea to dial the phone number for them yourself so you don't end up paying fifty dollars worth of international calls!

Recently, it has been discovered that telling them stories often sparks their imagination. These stories can be used as a catalyst for releasing thoughts that are trapped deep in the back of their minds collecting dust. You might ask, "Where does someone get such stories?" Well, remember the old saying about listening to your elders? Well, this is a perfect place to begin. If you're caring for a parent, the stories that were told to you throughout the years are ideal to recite back to them. These tales have special meanings to your loved ones. Even if you happen to tell a story wrong and get corrected, you have successfully induced a conversation. By knocking off the cobwebs from those pathways traveling through their brain, you may assist their mind in allowing them to tell you a story you never heard before.

Sadly, people suffering from dementia arrive at a point where they can no longer recall many of the facts about their own life, but they seem quite adept at constructing a new reality.

All of this takes a lot of energy, learning and patience. But you can enrich their lives by sharing the give and take, one story at a time. Learn to cherish the conversations you're now having, because when they are gone, trust me, they will truly be missed.

When they say things you know are wrong, learn not to correct them. This only puts them in a state of confusion. Also, keep your statements short and simple, but please don't demean them by speaking to them as if they are children.

If you're giving them instructions, only direct them to do one thing at a time. If you say to them, "You need to wash your hands and brush your teeth so we can go to the doctor," that will be too much for them to absorb. Mention one step at a time. You might even get out of the house sooner.

Eventually you'll start noticing that they won't stay on the same subject very long. They will stop in the middle of a sentence and then forget what they were saying. Pay close attention to their "body language." You'll soon learn their facial expressions like: pain, depression, confusion and love. They're all in there. Be patient and loving. It is as frustrating for them as it is for you, maybe more so.

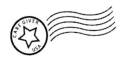

Dear Caregiver,

British merchant seaman Joseph Conrad, who later became a novelist, wrote: "No fear can stand up to hunger, no patience can wear it out."

One of your biggest battles as an Alzheimer's caregiver will be maintaining your loved ones' appetite.

GJL

Weight? I Just Ate

(Appetite, Swallowing and Constipation)

"I just ate an hour ago" was a proclamation I heard from Dad two or three times a week.

Malnutrition is a major concern in regards to an Alzheimer's patient and should always be on the caregiver's mind. Establishing a routine mealtime is a step that should be taken early on and remain throughout the course of the disease. Breakfast, lunch, and dinner, kept on a set schedule, helps keep things simple, therefore more bearable for a deteriorating mind.

Every evening, we had dinner at 6:30 p.m. This way when Dad went into his address about how he had already eaten, I would ask him to take a gander at his watch and remind him what time we always had supper. 'Nuff said.

Actually, sitting and eating together made meal-times go much smoother. Further, I never gave my father multiple choices for dinner. If I did, we would have had to reschedule dinner for 7:30 p.m. or later. Again simplicity is the rule.

The more confused Alzheimer's patients are before eating, the more often you will find large quantities of food left on their plates. If they protest that there's too much in front of them at the outset, you might try modest portions or even a smaller size plate.

Stick with whatever routine to which they're accustomed, whether it's a television broadcasting the news in the background or a quiet mellow atmosphere, if it works stick with it. Otherwise revert back to the old trial and error and eventually you'll find the right combination.

I'm once again advising you to pay close attention and learn as much as possible from your patient. Remembering his or her reactions will be your best teacher. In the long run it should noticeably ease stress for both of you.

At one point, my father had dropped ten pounds in a two-week period which could have been attributed to many different reasons. If this should happen to your loved one, it's important to apprise his or her physician immediately. Depression could very well be one of many contributing factors.

Don't assume the worst, but you should know this could be the advancement of the disease itself. Once again, pay close attention, especially to the patient's swallowing and speech.

Getting pills down will likely become a dilemma for you and your patient; if so, try using a thicker beverage to help push the medications down, something like tomato juice or even applesauce or ice cream. When swallowing pills, try having him or her keep the chin down against the chest, not facing up. Actually, looking up while swallowing will open the windpipe, but closes the esophagus, which is the complete opposite of what you want to do. This also helps to stifle a gag reflex.

"Ensure" or some other brand of high-calorie supplement might prove useful in helping to keep a pound or two on and supplying valuable nutrients.

A ground rule: Make sure your patient does not get constipated. Poison, due to constipation over a thirty-day blockage, nearly took my dad out. According to him, he was fine "two days ago." He kept repeating this as his health deteriorated. By the time we found out what was going on, his colon was completely obstructed and his body was full of toxins.

Don't rely on what an Alzheimer's victim is telling you. Somehow, constantly drill that into your head. You have to take matters into your own hands and make a judgment call, though heaven knows you have enough on your plate already.

New Beginnings

That first bright step into the sunshine of life
begins with the opening of the family cocoon.
The caterpillar becomes a butterfly
spreading her wings into the world.

What she is today is but a tiny mirror,
of the transformation that is yet to come.
For with time, love, humor and warmth
she is an ever changing masterpiece.

Whether as wife, mother, career woman or all,
she will find her center of peace.
A place that is hers and hers alone,
the essence of what she is and will be.

Using the instincts that each of us have
to find the good in each other,
to be a caring friend, lover, helper and playmate,
to listen and share, to laugh and cry.

With loving support of family and friends,
she takes flight down an unknown road towards her future,
like the rising of the sun in the east.
Each day filled with new beginnings.

Finding excitement and challenge at each new turn.
Her flight through life filled with many happy adventures
and memories to put in her book of life,
as the sun moves along that steady path across the sky.

When the sun at last begins to set in the west
and her flight nears its end, she can look back along her path
and know the she has been everything she can be
and has done her very best.

Esther Marie Latz

The Eyes of Alzheimer's

(Vision Problems)

If an Alzheimer's patient has a problem with their eyesight, their brain may be less adequate to compensate than a normal person due to the deterioration from the disease.

Any correctable vision should be addressed as early as possible because their memory impairment could be keeping them from recognizing what they're actually seeing. This condition is called *agnosia*—a loss of comprehension of vision, audio or other sensations.

Make an appointment with an ophthalmologist, advise the specialist that they have been diagnosed with Alzheimer's and need to have their eyes checked for any possible disorders.

If the patient has been wearing contact lenses, it's time to return to regular eyeglasses. The earlier you make the adjustment the better, and make sure you have at least one extra pair of glasses. These things have a way of walking off by themselves. Assign your-self the task of cleaning their glasses every morning. My father would swear his glasses were just fine, when actually they were so filthy, you might as well have been looking through a kaleidoscope.

It's best to keep the home well lit. I kept several lights on twenty-four hours a day for my dad. He slept in a bedroom which made me feel as if I should be spreading a layer of sunscreen all over myself. How-ever, the brightness kept him calm.

When you notice Alzheimer's patients shuffling their feet as they walk, often this is because their brains can't decipher what they're actually seeing in front of them, making them afraid to take that next step. En-tering into a room with a different colored carpet or tile might be interpreted as a step up or down.

A caregiver's main goal should be to relieve these people as much confusion as possible. If that means having their eyes checked annually or leaving a few extra lights on, I feel that's an extremely small price to pay.

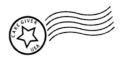

Dear Caregiver,

"A dream is a wish your heart makes, when you're fast asleep."
This was a plaque on the bedroom wall of my childhood; a sweet
sentiment to encourage calm slumber. Embrace it.

HBM

Bedtime

(Sleep Patterns and Caregiver's Respite)

As a caregiver of a person with Alzheimer's, you will find there are nights when your loved one just won't turn in for bed early enough. Soon, exhaustion has overwhelmed you. You're afraid to close your eyes because you just never know what could happen next.

People afflicted with Alzheimer's disease sometimes get their sleep patterns turned upside down. Caregivers run into a dilemma when their patients start sleeping later in the day. They don't want to wake them because it's probably the only peace and quiet they'll have all day, but the longer the patients sleep, the longer the day will last.

Their biological clock is ticking, but what if I were to tell you it doesn't keep the correct time anymore? This is basically what my dad's physician told me when

I asked, "How in the world can an eighty-five-year-old man stay awake for thirty hours straight, twice in one week?" His doctor explained that Dad no longer had any comprehension of time and during the latter stage of Alzheimer's it is common for these people to keep going for days.

What completely floored me was how my father could carry on for an entire day, sleep for only two hours and then wake up and start totally over. His routine practically killed me. I've learned to be a light sleeper from years of caregiving, but this excursion placed me into a full stage of exhaustion.

It was not only the fact that he was continuously awake, but he was also on the far side of restless, endlessly rubbing his hands, sitting down in a chair only to get back up within seconds, placing himself too often in harm's way. It got to the point where I was afraid to use the bathroom, terrified of what might happen during the few minutes I was away.

Even more perplexing was that the medications specifically prescribed to help him relax at night had zero effect. When your Alzheimer's patient has this condition, you both just have to ride it out.

I've heard horror stories of late-stage Alzheimer's patients staying awake for five whole days before meeting their Maker. Dad's physician helped remind me—all patients respond differently.

Hopefully, this won't happen in your situation. But, if it does, you'll have to pull out all your skills at caregiving, keeping their hands and fading mind constantly entertained for safety sake.

Use all outside assistance available. There's no reason to try to outlast them. It is improbable that you'll be able to keep up that pace for that long a cycle when it barely fazes them. You'll become a train wreck!

Make sure you use what hours of relief you get for solid REM sleep. You never know just how long the next ordeal could last.

When the sleep patterns of an Alzheimer's patient start to become disrupted, this is a strong indication that they are beginning to progress into another stage of the disease. And once sleep habits begin to be irregular throughout the night, there is an extremely pronounced chance that the patient will commence to wander. From this point on the dangers that lurk around every dark corner are countless. Right from the outset try to establish a solid routine for the time they awaken and the time they turn in for the night.

In the morning, expose these loved ones' bedrooms to as much sunlight as possible. This will help regulate their circadian cycle, also known as their biological clock. If the windows are not facing the east, get into the habit of turning on a bright overhead light, keeping the room well lit during their waking hours. Sunshine deficiency can play an enormous role in depression.

Another thing you might attempt is to avoid letting them take any daytime naps or at least limit it to one short catnap early on during the day.

Patients do well if they are engaged in both physical and mental activities daily, but do refrain from allowing them to become physical or exercise too close to their bedtime. And of course, keep them away from dietary stimulants such as sugar, caffeine and most kinds of junk food after evening hours. If they are in the earlier stages where they still have an appetite, try a light meal before bedtime, maybe with a warm glass of milk.

Talk to their physician to see if any of the medications they are consuming could be acting as a stimulant. Maybe they could take those only in the morning hours.

I had good results with giving my father about 6 mg of Melatonin every night with his dinner. This is an over-the-counter dietary supplement, which is made from the same natural ingredient that makes everyone sleepy after that Thanksgiving turkey dinner. We referred to it as "the turkey pill," and one nice feature is that it's easy to crush so it can be hidden in their food. However, I have talked to some caregivers who reported that it wasn't very effective on their loved ones. As I stated many times before, "Every patient responds differently."

But before trying any medication, whether over-the-counter or not, always confer with a doctor. He or she may want to prescribe something more potent or suggest something totally different. Unfortunately, I did experience that most medications that encourage sleep are not covered by Medicare and some other insurances.

A few years ago, I asked my dad's doctor to prescribe something to help him sleep. He was then getting in the habit of staying awake 'til 1:00-2:00 a.m., again it was just about killing me. Soon a problem with the pills became evident. They were affecting his balance and he was becoming dangerously unsteady. I feared he'd fall during a nightly trip to the bathroom, so within the first week, I decided to stop the pills, (That is until he finally digressed into the later stage of the disease.) Caregivers have to weigh the good and the bad; what worked yesterday and today might not work tomorrow.

Expect to perform a lot of trial and error in this regard. Keep in mind that it is important for patients to stay in a habitual sleep pattern. If they don't sleep, you won't either, and that's an unhealthy setting for both of you.

Many senior citizens are in the habit of enjoying a cup of coffee or tea after their evening dinner. Simply switch to a decaffeinated version. They don't have to know.

It's so important that the caregiver gets his or her share of rest. If you start your day already worn out, it will be a no-win situation. Call someone for respite sitting, at least for a couple of hours, so you can take a nap. It's that important.

In my father's case, one of the reasons he didn't want to go to bed was anxiety and nervousness. He developed a fear of being alone. If this happens, try sitting with them until they fall asleep. Unfortunately, once you start this, you might not be able to stop.

One of the main goals of every caregiver should be finding a way to have enough rest. Everything depends on it.

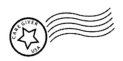

Dear Caregiver,

John D. Rockefeller was well known for his penny-pinching habits. While spending a winter in Florida, he went to a dentist to have a tooth pulled, "How much?" "Three dollars," the dentist replied. "Three dollars to remove a tooth! Here's a dollar, just loosen it a bit."

GJL

Oral Hygiene

The best advice I can give on the subject of oral hygiene is to have all dental needs attended to during the earliest onset of Alzheimer's. Toothaches or any other type of pain will only greatly contribute to the confusion.

While dealing with my father's Alzheimer's, I realized he had completely forgotten how to secure his dentures. As I would attempt to brush his teeth, he would clamp his jaw down so tight that you would think I was trying to break into Fort Knox! He was behaving as though I was about to extract all of his teeth. Whenever this occurred, I would simply brush the outside the best I could, coming back later for a more thorough cleaning at a more tranquil time. There's no reason to do battle about the matter. It will only make the situation worse.

I've constantly preached "routine" throughout my writings on caregiving for Alzheimer's patients. The subject of daily oral hygiene should be no different. There is no golden rule stating that their teeth have to be brushed first thing in the morning. Pick a time of day when they're most cooperative and stick to it.

Oral hygiene is extremely important for everyone's health and comfort. When patients' teeth hurt, they will probably just stop chewing. Since malnutrition is of special concern with Alzheimer's patients, the caregiver must be vigilant in order to avoid such a problem. It is a constant struggle to insure they are eating a sufficient diet.

Speak to the dentist and make sure he or she checks the patient thoroughly. One simply cannot rely on memory-impaired patients' responses when regarding discomfort.

Periodically check his or her gums for redness or sores.

Remember, Alzheimer's patients quickly forget about objects they can't see; out of sight, out of mind.

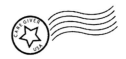

Dear Caregiver,

An unknown author wrote:"Simplicity is making the journey of this life with just baggage enough."

The simpler you make this journey for you and your loved one, the better both of you will fare.

GJL

The Closet of Simplicity

(Clothing)

As I've hammered from the beginning, "simple routine is number one in caring for people with Alzheimer's." This also applies in regards to their wardrobe. Keep it simple, as in loose fitting, easy to put on and take off. Also be sure to limit their choices, otherwise they will become overwhelmed and confused. There will be times when you wonder why they want to wear the same shirt every day; well, there might not be a yesterday belonging to their memory.

Let's start from the bottom-up. I had my dad wearing Velcro strap shoes. There was no reason to have him struggling to remember how to tie his shoes first thing in the morning, starting off his day in a frustrated state. The one thing I couldn't get him to wear was socks. I believe the cause of this was that he didn't want to wear anything tight, anywhere. I replaced his shoes fairly often so we could all breathe fresher surrounding air; I accomplished this identical shoe exchange in the middle of the night. He never knew the difference.

He liked to lay his pants across the foot of his bed at night. I'd also switch them out while he slept, replacing the belt and wallet making sure everything else went back into the proper pockets.

Shirts—loose fitting and comfort first. You might want to try bigger buttons or pullovers. Dad had a favorite flannel jacket that he wore through all four seasons. It had been washed so often it became velvety soft and was almost a security blanket for him. For a man that wore suit coats and ties all his life, it was surprising to see him settle into lumberjack attire.

Go with the flow. Pay attention to what the patients seem to prefer. It's vital for them to have a smooth start every morning. It could determine their level of confusion for the rest of the day or days to come. Once again, the "simple routine mind-set" can start with the simplicity of their closet and wardrobe.

Remember the Time and Place?

The chestnut man with the tranquil eye
ate a cold fig for his harvest pie
While his summer girl danced in the grain
distilling and echo, charming the sane

O, Lady, life is the dance of you
love is the dance with you
and deja vu ... is the dance we do

Yes, we were dancing in the street
but the time and place just had no feet

Peter Hanen

Patience is a Virtue

Patience is an essential ingredient for being a successful caregiver. In today's swift paced world, it's difficult to discipline oneself to slow down. Before I became my father's primary caregiver, I spent years working two jobs averaging thirteen hours a day, plus another two hours behind the wheel going to and fro. When I arrived in the world of caregiving, I felt as if I was constantly driving through a school zone! It was quite the culture shock.

When caring for a loved one with Alzheimer's, let yourself become part of their world, instead of trying to move them into yours.

I can't tell you how many mornings I spent trying to get my father ready for a doctor's appointment, finally asking myself, "Could he possibly be moving any slower?" On one occasion I decided he was trying to set a new Guinness Book World Record for the slowest shave. I was forever calling the doctor's office to inform them that we were running late as usual.

It takes a *patient* person to provide care when you're still able to move and process your thoughts quickly, but the person you're caring for cannot. It is understandably difficult to slow life down. I found myself constantly having to remind myself how important it was not to rush my father because all it ever accomplished was to increase his confusion tremendously.

Being an *impatient* caregiver will only fill the room with anxiety and fear for the both of you.

Keep your composure. It is not only important when they're moving in slow motion, but it also has much to do with keeping your cool while they're asking you the same question for the thirtieth time. Learning to bite your tongue and refrain from yelling "I just told you that" all falls into the same category: forbearance. If you catch yourself speaking in an angry voice, take a step outside and breathe in some fresh air and kick a little dirt around. You must remain diligent in your awareness of knowing when you're about to lose your patience. When you see this begin to happen more and more often, it's only common sense to recognize this as a sign that you are in dire need of some respite care.

Patience is the state of endurance under extremely trying circumstances, and there's no better example of these circumstances than when caregiving.

I don't know who first said, "Patience is a virtue," but I believe they might have been a caregiver at one point in their life.

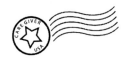

Dear Caregiver,

Motivational speaker, author and super salesperson Zig Ziglar once said: "People often say that motivation doesn't last. Well, neither does bathing—that's why we recommend it daily."

Daily or not, bathwater definitely wears off.

GJL

Bath Time

(Bathing with Dignity)

Feelings of pride, dignity and embarrassment loom large in the matter of bathing Alzheimer's patients. Between the self-consciousness and loss of independence, this task must be handled with utmost compassion.

If you're familiar with their already established daily routine, try to continue to follow that pattern. My father was one who first ate breakfast, then shaved and showered. I learned how much more difficult it was to bathe him in the evenings, always telling me how he had already washed that morning.

As I have said, it's best to keep all Alzheimer's patients in a daily routine. You'll run into the situation where they might have an early morning doctor's appointment. The chances of your arriving on time are extremely slim if you plan on bathing them that morning. There's enough time-killing procrastination going on already. These are times when bathing in the evening might work to your advantage.

Here are some suggestions on how to preserve Alzheimer's patients' privacy: Place a large towel or robe over their shoulders and one over their lap and then try washing under the towel. It's important to have bathing items ready and laid out so you won't have to stop and leave the patients unattended during the middle of the procedure. Never leave them alone. It only takes a microsecond for something bad to happen. Install whatever safety devices are needed: handrails, traction strips, shower bench and a handheld shower sprayer; these are a must for proper rinsing. I'm sure you know how to prepare the basics: water temperature, towels and shampoo. Try sticking to the same brands. They will get accustomed to certain aromas.

There are ways to softly coax them into bathing. Tell them you would like to wash their back, "Please remove your shirt." Once their shirt is off say, "I'd like to wash your feet. Is it okay if I take your shoes off?" Keep up this approach until you finally have them in their birthday suit.

There will be good days and bad days. If you're upsetting them too much, you might want to bring into play the old-fashioned sponge bath. You don't want to overstress the issue. If the experience becomes too dramatic, it might be even more difficult the next time.

Please, do not tell them they stink. This is an approach they'll only find offensive and will get you absolutely nowhere. Nobody likes to be insulted, even if it's true.

Bathing them two or three times a week should be sufficient unless they become incontinent. Then you'll have to wash and observe their skin condition daily. Make sure pressure sores don't arise and become infected. If you notice any area you're worried about, contact their physician right away.

Try to make their bathing experience as pleasurable as possible. It's best to have the same person do all the bathing rather than different faces. Keep to the same routine as much as possible. There will be times when they flat-out refuse. As the caregiver, you must be flexible; an hour or two later might bring totally different results.

Dear Caregiver,

One of the many dedicated support group leaders is Karen Francis. She tells her caregivers, "One of my rules to remember is that ice cream solves everything!"

GJL

Bedsores

(Pressure Sores or Decubitus Ulcers)

When a person ages, the skin becomes thinner. Thus, when some elderly people become bedridden, bedsores, also known as pressure sores or decubitus ulcers occur easily. These sores result from sustained pressure to a body area which prevents normal blood flow. Without adequate circulation the impaired skin dies.

The severity of pressure sores can be observed in four distinct stages. Stage one is where the wound is an irritated red patch of skin that usually dissipates after a short period of time once the pressure is relieved. The irritation can become worse until finally reaching the fourth stage, which results in a large area of skin loss, possibly damaging the muscle and even bone.

Such sores can be a caregiver's nightmare and cause unimaginable suffering to their dear loved one.

While taking care of my father, we battled this dilemma daily throughout the last couple of years of his life; the less mobile he became, the more attention I had to pay to his skin condition.

If your patient is wheelchair-bound, you may think your only concern will be bedsores on his or her bottom. But in fact, you will also need to pay close attention to the shoulder blades, the spine and the back of their arms. If bedbound, you also need to keep an eye on their ears and along the back and sides of their head, actually any point where the body pressure occurs.

Prevention will always be a caregiver's best defense. Examining the skin while bathing should become a daily ritual. Once he or she has become incontinent, your constant vigil becomes even more critical. The skin staying moist only enhances the risk of bedsores creating a higher contingency of infection.

If sores become open, they can take forever to heal. They must be attended to every day. Your loved ones' doctor can design a plan for you to follow, but the first step of treating any bedsore is to relieve any pressure that caused it. If they cannot reposition themselves, someone will have to turn them throughout the entire day possibly up to every two hours. Be sure to watch out for things like wrinkled sheets, the plastic of incontinence pads or any materials that could be restricting circulation.

Current technology has brought forward some great devices to assist with patient care; air or water-filled cushions, specialized mattresses, skin care salves and many other helpful products. See if you can get some of these products prescribed by the attending physician as most insurance policies will cover the cost. One rule that should always be followed is to contact his or her doctor immediately if you notice the sore had broken open. This is where the wound becomes extremely vulnerable to infection.

When visiting loved ones in a nursing home or hospital, don't hesitate to check their skin. If anything concerns you, talk with a member of the nursing staff or the facility director. Inform them you'll be back daily and will faithfully check on their condition.

During my father's final days, it seemed no matter how often we turned him; we couldn't prevent his skin from breaking down. It's a tough and heartbreaking battle. Just show up every day and do the best you can.

Nothing Is Impossible

On an evening in '57 you could watch a new star
Hear a new sound from the sky
That tiny Russian basketball,
And then in '69 you could watch an Eagle land
Hear one small step
That US moonwalk in the night

In '04 before the great war
Outside scifi none saw those events ahead,
And most take as given all they've got
Though progress is a dicey proposition.

This '04 a man we knew, knew that well,
sliced boundaries to ribbons,
Flew against odds,
To keep the progress coming.

No cathedrals bear his name, and we've
No sacred texts to read
No candles to light in alcoves,
No hymns to sing for him

Yet for those in greatest peril,
Those in greatest pain,
Those who fight in battle,
He still is here all ways

For them, for us, for the many and the few,
He would open any cell,
Stem any tide,
Ride down all the wind's dark eyes,
Any night and every day ...

May you say hello to Krypton for us.
We miss you Christopher Reeves.

For Christopher Reeves

(September 25, 1952–October 10, 2004)

Peter Hanen

Incontinence

(Cleanup and Incontinence Products)

Caregivers need to realize they're not handling biohazardous material here. I know most people become squeamish when dealing with human waste. But caring for people who are incontinent is a learning process; like everything else a caregiver endures.

Almost 100 percent of Alzheimer's patients will arrive at a point where they lose control of their bladder and/or bowels, most likely both. At this stage of the disease, most families are usually advised that the time has come to institutionalize their loved ones. Even so, countless families continue caring for them at home until their final days.

Incontinence begins with some occasional accidents, possibly because they couldn't make it to the bathroom quickly enough or were unable to remove their clothing in time. I learned to dress my father with pants that had an elastic waistband; pull up, pull down, quick and easy.

It's important to help them preserve as much dignity as possible. Train yourself to say things like, "Oh, you spilled something on your pants," rather than, "Oh my! I see you had another accident."

Think of Ronald Reagan and Christopher Reeves. One was the U.S. President and the other Superman. These were the very essence of people of dignity. However, the need for adult diapers became necessary but in no way detracted from their honor and respectability.

Incontinence pads, adult diapers, and other such health-care products are intended to keep patients' bottoms clean and protected along with furniture, clothing, and other consequential yet replaceable objects. Keep in mind you're crossing the personal barrier of self-respect. However, as the caregiver, it has to be your decision when to start using these products. Incontinence care is more difficult with Alzheimer's patients because of their inability to make right choices. They may for instance suddenly rip their nappies off, not understanding why they are suddenly wearing such an item.

In the event you may wish to include them on an outing, keep a bag packed at all times containing clothing, wipes and any of the incontinence products you may find necessary.

The dreaded fear of the cleanup is far worse than the actual task. Once you get past that squeamish point, the routine becomes easier. Keep things organized; put everything in one convenient place so you will not need to dash out of the room in the middle of a cleaning, only to return, finding a mess every-where.

Keep a daily record of the time of day they urinate or have a bowel movement. This way you'll learn when they should be seated on the toilet.

Also, be sure to pay close attention to their skin as a little redness can quickly develop into a nasty bed-sore.

Lastly, make sure you have latex gloves that fit. By the time you finally get those darn things on, you could be dealing with pure chaos!

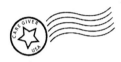

Dear Caregiver,

"To the world you might be one person, but to one person you might be the world." This was written by an unknown author, but I can only imagine it is exactly what loved ones are thinking about the one person who is staying by their side; their caregiver, their world, you.

GJL

Reflections of Alzheimer's

(The Trouble with Mirrors)

Trying to wash or shave a loved one with Alzheimer's will eventually become extremely difficult as the disease advances. One culprit that could be playing a role in such difficulties is a mirror. This may sound crazy, but your loved one might believe that there is a stranger in the room staring at him or her, thus causing a refusal to get undressed until that reflection leaves or at least closes its eyes.

I read about a man with Alzheimer's who actually began stashing food for the unidentified person because he felt no one was feeding him. As bizarre as that sounds, I can relate to such an incident after taking care of my father for so many years. We had a full-length mirror in our bathroom which made my dad suspicious of his own image. He began wanting to only shave at our kitchen sink, using the window almost as a reflector and finally only seated at the kitchen table, using a small cosmetic mirror.

Imagine in your mind's eye that you are still in your early twenties. You wake up one morning, look in the mirror and suddenly you see yourself as an eighty-year-old man or woman. You would truly become overwhelmed seeing yourself having aged sixty years overnight or appalled that a stranger got into your house. Clearly, this is not a good way for an Alzheimer's patient to begin the day.

Often my father would ask at bedtime if he had school in the morning. When he went to bed believing he was a child, he would most likely awaken with the same thought still imbedded in his head.

This is one situation that as a caregiver, you have some control over. Cover or remove all mirrors in the living area. Keep a portable one handy for your personal use and for times that you feel are appropriate for them.

Not all patients see reflections as threatening or unconversant. Some actually befriend their new image and try to communicate with it.

Stick to the ground rule of trial and error. If they start to get upset for no obvious reason, it may be merely a perception that an uninvited guest has invaded their home.

I'm Always Me

Look at me
What do you see?
I've changed from years ago
But I'm still me.

When I am scared
I may cry, I may wander
reassure me, talk to me.

When I'm cold or hungry
I may holler, act restless,
let me know I'm safe
explain these things to me.

Even when I'm frustrated
Strike out at any one near
I need you to guide me
Comfort and love me.
Because I'm still me.

Esther Marie Latz

Shadowing

Shadowing is the act of an Alzheimer's or dementia victim attempting to keep his or her caregiver in sight at all times.

In caring for my father, there were times when I didn't even have to turn around. I could feel the warmth of my father's breath heating up the back of my neck. He would constantly follow me around like a small child clinging to its mother's dress.

Even if I left him with a respite caregiver for an hour or two, he would perpetually ask where I was, sometimes more than twenty times in a half hour. This could obviously drive the person staying with him almost to the point of madness. This behavior began right around the same time he began showing signs of sundowner's (sundown syndrome).

There is a lot of fear involved for someone who is suffering from being memory impaired. People living with Alzheimer's can experience this all day long. They finally get to a stage where they just don't feel safe alone anymore. I've always said, "Controlling their anxiety is half the battle."

Their primary caregiver becomes a security blanket, a lifeline, the center of their world, and they want to always be with them, following them everywhere and I mean everywhere! Bathrooms included. Sometimes even mimicking them; it becomes really unsettling and extremely tiresome.

When this conduct begins, try to recognize what time of day it happens the most. This will give you a notion of when to find a repetitious activity to keep them entertained. Consider asking them to help fold some laundry or work on a hobby they always loved such as a jigsaw puzzle or playing solitaire.

Also, I can't tell you how many times I woke up to find my dad just staring at me, watching me sleep or actually waking me up just to ask if I was sleeping.

Shadowing is just one of the myriads of symptoms Alzheimer's victims go through, but for the caregiver, it can definitely be one of the more unnerving ones.

Dear Caregiver,

A man with Alzheimer's told his wife, "I don't know how you ever expect me to remember your birthday when you never look a day older."

It would be awfully hard to get mad at him for forgetting after that!

GJL

What Happened to It?

(Hoarding)

"I just put it down here a minute ago. It has to be here." This is something you'll have to become used to hearing while being a caregiver to a loved one with Alzheimer's.

You may soon find that loved ones have developed a habit of hoarding or collecting things. They have hiding places so secretive that you'll wish you had thought of them. Dad loved to hoard any book he could grab. You have to learn to go with the flow of things. This may keep them at ease.

My father had a pile of books stacked where he always sat at our kitchen table. If it comforted him to eat surrounded by books, so be it. Eventually, I had to install a shelf along the wall at the table so we'd have enough room for two dinner plates, and still be able to see each other.

He and I had been booksellers for seventeen years, so these were items from which he took comfort and also things he could relate to, especially the pricing of them. I had even found our local Yellow Pages priced, ready for sale. So if I found myself missing a book I just had in my hands, there was a 95 percent chance it had become part of his collection.

I hate to say this, but if you're caring for a person with Alzheimer's, a time will come when you'll have to lock certain cabinets or drawers in order to protect and preserve important possessions.

Once, I spent several days checking every crack and crevice throughout our house searching for my missing wallet. When asking Dad over and over if he had seen my billfold, I repeatedly received the same reply, "no." I finally asked him to stand up. While "patting him down," I found my black one in his left back pocket and his brown one in his right.

I know you're thinking that I should have used common sense and checked his pockets first, but you have to be sensitive in how you handle things. I simply put my newly rediscovered wallet back in my pocket and told him, "They look almost identical," patted him on his back and left the matter alone, never to be mentioned again.

Try not to upset Alzheimer's patients. They are always a hair away from massive depression. They're storing so much sorrow inside their souls that if they could stash all that emotion, they'd need a bigger hiding place.

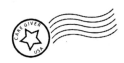

Dear Caregiver,

Alzheimer's patients will go through a stage where they suspect everybody is up to something. American social writer and philosopher Eric Hoffer wrote: "The suspicious mind believes more than it doubts."

Being a caregiver, you must learn not to take any accusations personally. It's all part of the disease.

GJL

Suspicious Minds

(Accusations of Stealing and Adult Day Care)

One of the problems I found with using a babysitter (and how I truly detest using that word) is that Dad always believed that the sitter was stealing everything he owned.

It's a blistering experience for caregivers and family members to endure, especially after devoting their entire heart and soul to helping their loved ones to cope with Alzheimer's; suddenly they are falsely accused of stealing. It can range from a small personal item to everything the person owns!

In many cases, people suffering from Alzheimer's and other dementia-related diseases will exhibit symptoms of paranoid delusions. This often comes directly from having all the decisions about how they live now made for them, making them feel no longer in control.

There may be times when the ones we are caring for actually surrender a favorite item of theirs and within moments they become frantic, making accusations about the item being stolen along with everything else they believe is missing. This dilemma may accelerate to the point where it might be wise not to accept any more gifts. I suggest keeping the object only until a chance arises to sneak it back into place.

Much of the time what is truly occurring is that they're hiding everything in their secret hiding spots, quickly forgetting where they put them. Then once again caregivers find themselves accused of being kleptomaniacs.

If this happens, you may spend hours searching through the entire house for whatever they misplaced and throughout the whole time you have to listen to the accusation of what a horrible person you are. If they could only realize you barely have a minute for yourself as it is. There's certainly not any time to waste thinking up plots against them!

It's extremely hard not to take these accusations personally. After a while, you even start feeling a bit guilty.

Try expressing how you understand the importance of their belongings and that you would never take or move anything without asking first.

Another problem you may run into is that when you take them shopping, quite a few items end up in their pockets. Suddenly the shoe is on the other foot and they're the ones accused of stealing. Ask their attending physician to prepare a letter, stating that they have been diagnosed with dementia. Always keep this note available in case you run into trouble with store security. You also may want to consider dressing them in clothing without pockets. Remember, "Idle hands are the devil's toys."

My father would have a one-hour conversation with his sitting companion, leave to go to the bathroom only to return shouting, "What the heck are you doing in my house?" Being a friend of the family did not matter. Suspicion led him into thinking they were always talking about him behind his back.

Dad treated one sitter with such an abrupt attitude that he would only address her as, "babysitter," yet, at that time, I believed he knew her first name very well. During such bouts, someone will undoubtedly be falsely accused and feelings will be hurt. It's inevitable.

There are day care centers specializing in adult supervision, some suited to special needs for Alzheimer's patients. I believe this could be a plus during the early stages of the disease. Hopefully, if you start them early enough, they may adapt and make friends. This could enable you, the caregiver, to continue to hold down an outside job and bring home some much needed finances.

But after the disease progresses, they might become more combative or verbally abusive. Wandering, trying to get themselves home could become another concern; these are problems that the day care center might not accept nor employ properly trained staff to handle. It only takes one in the group to act out and the confusion could spread like wildfire.

Although every Alzheimer's patient responds differently, these centers may be worth a try if you can persuade your loved one to accept the idea. Forcing matters will only turn into a catastrophe.

A prominent part of the problem lies with patients feeling degraded from the loss of their independence. Continue to keep reassuring them they will never be left alone.

Dear Caregiver,

Saint Francis of Assisi, founder of the Franciscans, once said: "A single sunbeam is enough to drive away many shadows."

You will learn, as the caregiver of an Alzheimer's patient, the importance of light.

GJL

Don't Turn Off the Light

(Keeping Things Well Lit)

While my dad's Alzheimer's progressed, he insist-
ed on sleeping with a light on in his room. I'm not
talking about a night light, but one bright enough to
read a pocket-size dictionary. Having his room glar-
ingly illuminated made it easier for him to calculate
his surroundings. After all, Alzheimer's patients are
likely to start their day off not realizing whose house
they're even in.

I placed family photos along the wall beside Dad's
bed. This was to familiarize and comfort him when he
first opened his eyes. Photo albums are a great tool
to have lying around the home of an Alzheimer's patient. My dad spent hours flipping through the pages
of these old photographs; not always remembering
the faces from his past but somehow definitely receiving solace during times of confusion.

Even after waking from a catnap in his recliner, it became difficult for him to get his bearings.

Try not to change patients' surroundings. Redecorating their home or changing an art piece on the wall can severely disorient them.

I recall an incident where Dad asked me why someone removed the bed from his room. The only change made was clean sheets and a different colored heavier blanket. Minor changes that would normally seem innocuous could send him into a state of confusion. It even caused hallucinations. So keep things simple and well lit. The memory impaired need their familiar surroundings to remain unchanged.

Holding On

Life can change forever in a day
the sky once bright is now dark and grey
This man I knew has gone away
and another man is here to stay
He's in the shadow of a man gone by
no matter how long or hard I try
It shows in the silence of his eye
his youth and strength do not apply.

Esther Marie Latz

Sundown Syndrome

(Sundowning and Evening Confusion)

Around 4:45 p.m.—everyone gets a new name, possibly two. My father, who didn't seem to need a clock for this, went through this change daily toward the end of the moderate stage of Alzheimer's disease.

Sundown syndrome—also known as "sundowning"—is a term describing the onset of heavier confusion and intensified agitation. Usually, this begins anywhere from late afternoon to dusk. In reality, it could happen anytime throughout the day.

Experts believe one of the contributing factors is a shift in the biological clock, caused from the change of daylight to dark. Keeping the house well lit during these hours will help immensely.

Physical and mental exhaustion is one of the biggest culprits. An Alzheimer's patient's day consists of coping with who's who, "where am I," and living in the past. This would mentally drain anyone.

Once again, routine is the most helpful thing for your memory-impaired loved one. Evening hours usually become the busiest in a household; people coming and going, cooking supper, phone calls and the list goes on. If the traffic in your home is high volume, try placing them in a quieter room.

There were days when I swore my father's sundowners would last morning 'til night. I also recall noticing similar reactions on dispiriting rainy days. Once anxiety builds, it's difficult to turn it around. Keep evenings as calm, routine and simple as possible. Just do the best you can.

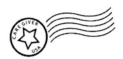

Dear Caregiver,

British poet and novelist Oliver Goldsmith wrote: "On the stage he was natural, simple, affecting; Twas only when he was off the stage he was acting."

As a caregiver, you will find yourself on stage more often than not as the Alzheimer's advances.

GJL

Role Playing

(Adapting to Character)

You will discover, as the disease of Alzheimer's progresses, everyone that your loved one knows may receive a new identity; names might change five times or more in a one-hour period.

There is no way to prepare yourself ahead of time for the jarring moment when your loved one looks at you and has no recognition of who you are—it's nothing short of heartbreaking!

There will be moments when, suddenly, he or she will comprehend who you actually are, but these occasions are becoming few and far between. When those moments do occur, you will observe through their facial expressions, the profound sorrow he or she feels.

You must accept that it's not their fault. Pursue the role they believe you to be and assume your new identity. First, you usually become a close relative; brother, sister, uncle, aunt or family member deep from the past. Later you will assume still another role; names seem to be randomly drawn out of a hat.

My father most often believed I was his dad. I learned to make this work to my advantage. He definitely listened to me with deeper respect. He would ask, "Dad, do I have to take all these pills?" and then I would softly respond, "Yes son, please take them all and don't make me get your mother involved." Playing the role can help both parties. I had become Dad 80 percent of the time, brothers and who knows who 15 percent. Being recognized as his son dwindled to a diminishing final 5 percent.

My father, being the oldest of seventeen children in his family would constantly ask for his brother, Alfie, who was the second eldest. Well the reality is, Alfie had passed away shortly after World War II. If I even attempted to tell him this, he would become extremely upset, yelling, "How could you people not even tell me about my brother's funeral? I can't believe I missed it." I learned just to reflexively tell him, "Alfie just left. He said something about he'd be back in the morning."

Go with the flow. Caregiving is extremely demanding when this happens, but by playing along with the current scenario, you will be instrumental in comforting and relieving some of the stress. You must learn to quickly adapt—they did.

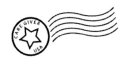

Dear Caregiver,

William Shakespeare wrote something that really coincides with the next story. He wrote: "The voice of parents is the voice of gods, for to their children they are heaven's lieutenants."

GJL

Voice of Authority

(Household Management and Stern Reasoning)

There will be many situations when a caregiver must decide what role to play. It can become awkward being the guardian, especially when one is caring for a parent. But that's exactly the role that must be assumed. While being my father's caregiver for a decade, I experienced a plethora of times when I felt uneasy using a voice of authority toward him. I'm not speaking about scolding him, just using a voice of stern reason.

This behavior triumphs over the rule I was taught from a young age—"Respect your elders!" Dealing with Alzheimer's patients who have reached a senior status necessitates that you assume the right to disregard that golden etiquette mandate.

As a caregiver, prepare for your time to be monopolized. One reason you need to be constantly by their side is that they are no longer able to make adult decisions; therefore, it is acceptable using a parental voice—within reason.

Safety is a top priority. If using a voice of authority redirects a patient from wandering out the front door without resulting in an anxiety attack—you did the right thing.

Usually the primary caregiver runs the whole household, becoming a business manager as well. When you, yourself take on the responsibilities as if you were running a business, it is not a bad way to go about things. Learn to write everything down and make a schedule devoting certain times to care for unavoidable tasks. If you're paying any of the household bills, electronic checking is a blessing. Automatic payments might keep you from sitting in the dark. Trust me, the electric company doesn't care that you've been sitting by a loved ones' side twenty-four hours a day and that's why you simply forgot to mail a check.

According to research, there are two kinds of caregivers; the one that can accept the situation and the second kind that has trouble adapting. Surveys show that nonadapters deal with patients that experience a higher level of hyperactivity. I've always believed Alzheimer's patients feed off their caregiver's emotions. The smoother the household runs, the easier it will be to keep up a positive, calm demeanor. Even so, there'll always be moments when everything feels like it's falling apart.

Listen to your own inner voice of authority and brush those other moments aside. Cling to the simplicities; things have a way of sorting themselves out.

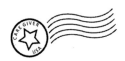

Dear Caregiver,

Learn to brush off any insults that patients may throw at you. There's a good chance that they don't even realize who you are at that particular moment.

Actress Bette Davis once said: "If you have never been hated by your child, you have never been a parent."

Dealing with Alzheimer's, often you will switch roles and become the parent.

GJL

Raging Fury

(Verbal Abuse, Frustration and Anxiety)

Memory-impaired patients may oftentimes exhibit a full spectrum of wrath and fury toward you, the caregiver: screaming accusations, throwing objects and calling you spiteful names.

Obviously this will become upsetting, but remember, this rage of hostility is not specifically directed at you. Usually, it is set in motion from overwhelming frustration because suffering from Alzheimer's or other dementia-related diseases will wear a patient down.

Studies reveal that most anger and frustration is generated from anxiety. For instance, asking patients to perform a task as simple as shaving may trigger a verbal confrontation and it could be that at this particular moment they might not remember how, responding with a straight out "No!" Broaching the subject too soon again could possibly send them into another rage.

It is easier for patients to refuse than to allow themselves to look foolish.

Get into the habit of redirecting your patient's thoughts, preferably to more blithesome ones. Try saying, "Remember the old days?" or "I love the color of that sweater." Train yourself to apply this technique during the many challenging situations you will encounter; life just might flow a little more smoothly.

I've never been one to push medications, but at this stage in Alzheimer's patients' lives, they are probably already consuming a bowlful each day. Talking to their physician about prescribing something for anxiety won't hurt.

There is a lot of fear involved for someone who is suffering from being memory impaired. I always kind of analyzed it like this; if you went to the mall to do some shopping and upon walking outside, you suddenly realize you have no idea where you parked your car, well, this wave of anxiety starts washing over you—it's terrifying and paralyzing. In a similar way, persons living with Alzheimer's experience this all day long.

One positive aspect of having no short-term memory is that a couple of minutes down the road, they won't even remember being upset.

Redirecting them on to different subjects is your best strategic defense. Train yourself to keep this as a communication standard and hopefully a couple of minutes later they are liable to have forgotten the entire episode anyway.

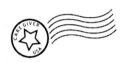

Dear Caregiver,

Viktor Frankl, a holocaust survivor and author of best seller, "Man's Search for Meaning," wrote: "When we are no longer able to change a situation … We are challenged to change ourselves."

As a caregiver, you will be challenged endlessly. Keep Frankl's advice in mind.

GJL

Redirection

(Trying to Avoid Frustration and Anxiety)

When my father progressed into the last stage of Alzheimer's, redirecting his thoughts became almost impossible.

Previously, I was able to turn his fixation on to a different subject, but in the final stage his delusions and hallucinations became so pronounced that I could only divert his train of thought for a few seconds at best.

When caring for an Alzheimer's patient, you must learn to use redirection to your advantage. Knowing just when confusion is beginning to snowball straight into delusion and using simply phrased words can create a U-turn in his or her thought patterns. These are skills you need to master.

When the afflicted patient begins speaking of a topic which makes absolutely no sense, casually interrupt with a quick question like, "That color looks great on you. Do you enjoy wearing that shirt?"

Steering the patient's mind on to a subject he or she can actually see, smell or touch will save hours of misery having to listen to meaningless chatter. Try handing them a couple of items like two different colored wash cloths; for example, a green one and a blue one. Ask them which of the two they like better. It may be an hour before you get an answer or maybe never. The point is you now have directed their confused thoughts on to another subject.

If they are still able to chew and swallow, you might want to try something referred to as "Gum Therapy." It's worth a try. A single stick of chewing gum might land you a peaceful thirty minutes.

Anxiety could be playing a significant role in causing severe disorientation. If the patient has already been on a particular anxiety medication for a long period of time, it might be beneficial to discuss with his or her physician the possibility of increasing the dosage or trying something new. I was against medicating my father at first. However, as symptoms of the disease advanced, I soon realized the blessing of palliative care.

Many of my father's mornings began with him believing he was on a train. He would ask, "Could you please tell me when the next stop is going to be? I believe that's where I have to get off." When I tried to reassure him that we were home in our own house, his response was, "Come on! I can feel the train moving." It's best to just go along with the ride. The last thing

I needed was to get his feathers all ruffled before his day even started.

So Dear Caregivers, hold on tight. From here on out, the ride will have fewer stops. Certain memories that drift through the patients' minds just won't float away anymore. If a mental image has worked them into a frenzy, chances are it's going to last the entire day. One of the hardest things I dealt with was convincing my father he was home. He constantly wanted to know why he could not go to his parents' house or some other place that he believed was his abode.

All during the last stage of the disease, as you care for your loved one at home, you'll probably need the minimum of two people. Attempting to do everything yourself could erupt into a physical or mental fiasco, probably both. Create a schedule so that you know when relief is coming.

If our loved ones were able, they would surely advise us to take care of ourselves, so that when the inevitable comes to pass and they die, we will hopefully be able to begin enjoying our own lives again.

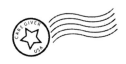

Dear Caregiver,

I'm sorry to tell you this, but there will undoubtedly be times when your loved ones will try your patience and their stubborn behavior will be the rule of the day!

As you rise above the situation, and you will, remember this: "A stubborn horse walks behind you, an impatient horse walks in front of you, but a noble companion walks beside you."

Choose nobility!

HBM

I Already Did It

(Stubbornness)

A good example of stubbornness from Alzheimer's patients can materialize from a visit to the doctor. Between his nervousness and anxiety, it was difficult to motivate my father. We were lucky to make it to an appointment at all.

When Alzheimer's patients refuse to do something, it's probably because it is less embarrassing for them to refuse, rather than to attempt and risk failing a simple task. Being uncooperative may be easier for them than looking foolish. Keep in mind that their attitude may very well be induced by the brain impairment caused by the disease.

Now, if patients are stubborn prior to the development of Alzheimer's, the caregiver's hands will likely be extra full. Most characteristics stay with them throughout the course of the disease.

Here are some common excuses:

- · I already did that
- · I'll do it later
- · I don't want to
- · I don't have time

Don't take these remarks personally.

Nobody likes to look foolish. If patients are being stubborn, try asking them again to do whatever task is at hand, making certain that only the two of you are present. Things might flow a little smoother. There will be times when it doesn't matter what you say or do. Never force an issue to the point of argument, just let the dust die down and try again later.

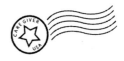

Dear Caregiver,

There is an old Spanish proverb that goes: "The busy man is troubled with but one devil, the idle man by thousands."

GJL

Idle Hands

(Activities for People
with Alzheimer's)

While caring for loved ones with Alzheimer's always remember this: *Idle hands are the devil's toys,* especially in the later stages of the disease.

It's necessary to keep them occupied. Place a photo album, playing cards, magazines in front of them, anything to keep them entertained. Keep their confused minds as absorbed as possible—before they attempt to do it themselves. This will lower the risk of them getting hurt.

Carefully chosen activities may help to keep our loved ones' anxieties to a minimum. It may also assist in diverting them from other behavioral problems created by Alzheimer's, aiding them to continue to have creative meaning in their lives. It's important for them to have a sense that they're still useful and a vital part of their families.

Keeping them active may or may not slow down the progression of the disease. What it will accomplish is to prolong the ability of their motor skills to continue to function. The fact that they're still working with their hands will help immensely in the battle to maintain coordination, which will only improve their quality of life.

Try venturing into hobbies that they enjoyed in the past. Continue to guide them in practicing their skills, tailoring each activity as the disease progresses, making certain that your expectations are not exceeding their abilities. This careful monitoring could prevent a wave of anxiety from washing over them, leaving them submerged in confusion. If a favorite activity includes game pieces or other articles, you may find that as the disease moves forward, switching to larger objects which will be easier for them to manipulate and also harder for them to swallow.

Always have a safe work area that is well lit and also a backup project on hand, just in case they become too frustrated with what they are currently working on.

Including patients in simple and familiar household duties can be wonderful as they leave them with a positive feeling that they are still needed. Try a basket full of laundry to fold or maybe a box of mixed up socks. Having them sort things is usually a success. Make a point of telling them how helpful they are being and remind them often of what an enormous favor it is to you when they help.

Crafts are always a great choice. Take knitting for example, even if they don't knit, simply having them roll all that yarn into a ball might work. There is something about repetition that creates a calming effect.

Be creative; make a jigsaw puzzle out of a copy of a family photograph. Try something that may have some personal meaning to them. It may even inspire a little conversation along the way.

Here is a surprising possibility; they may now have more of a budding artist in them than you would think! This is because they may no longer be as critical about the work they do. Watercolors, drawing, even creating a scrapbook may be something they now enjoy doing. Of course, this is all trial and error. They are still unique individuals.

Don't forget about the great outdoors. If they were once interested in gardening this might be perfect. It's always good for them, and for you, to get some exercise and fresh air, but you will have to make sure they are supervised and don't wander off or get themselves into any unwarranted mischief.

Most importantly, don't fret. There are all sorts of resources, including Googling "Alzheimer's Activities." I was amazed at the amount of Websites that popped up. One site even listed "101 things to do with an Alzheimer's person."

Help in dealing with this tragic disease has certainly come a long way.

When it comes to mealtime, my advice is: have something interesting already on the table in arm's reach; a newspaper, crafts, anything since you now have them sitting; keep their attention flowing. It's when they're idle that trouble brews.

This may sound as if I'm speaking of watching a small child. I detest admitting it, but there's an abundance of similarities. Just please, don't treat or speak to them in a childlike manner; they deserve more.

Accidents happen in microseconds. You can't be there for every single one. Keeping their hands busy, especially before you leave the room is a great rule to follow—might even help prevent a trip to the emergency room.

Dear Caregiver,

Are you searching for balance? Well, so is your loved one; both physical balance, with the use of a cane or walker, and emotional balance when learning to trust you as their best friend.

Tell them over and over:

"Lean on me, when you're not strong,
I'll be your friend. I'll help you carry on."

Yes, we all need someone to lean on.

HBM

Walkabout

(Balance and Safety Devices)

My dad's walking skills declined with the progression of Alzheimer's. He had a walker that helped support his balance, but he all too often forgot owning one and kept spontaneously getting up without it.

When Alzheimer's patients begin to frequently lose their balance or you notice their steps becoming shuffled, talk to their physician. There might be other medical reasons for this. Medications or other physical complications could be contributing factors.

This is when it becomes important to have the house safely arranged. Dispose of all throw rugs. Walkways should be well lit. Pay close attention to places at which they hesitate or avoid. Chairs with sturdy arms will help them push themselves to their feet. I had an empty frame of a commode strapped over our toilet so my dad could help raise and steady himself. One fall could take years away from a patient's longevity. A physical therapist can teach you techniques that will help prevent both of you from getting hurt.

Incorrect shoes could also be a dangerous factor: avoid slick soles, untied laces and heels that could catch on something like a threshold. I had my father in shoes with Velcro straps, eliminating shoestrings altogether. Slippers might be comfortable, but if they come off in midstride—just the confusion could quickly cause an accident.

Once again, you have to observe patients closely. See if you notice anything causing them to struggle. Sometimes just minor changes in the home can prevent a major disaster.

Dear Caregiver,

John Ruskin, art critic and author said something that is well worth every caregiver pondering: "The highest reward for a person's toil is not what they get for it, but what they become by it."

Once you make it through this noble campaign of caring, you will undoubtedly look at life differently; mostly because now you will have a newfound appreciation for everything.

GJL

Losing Sense of Time

Usually, it's difficult to notice when Alzheimer's patients progress from the early stage of the disease into the moderate phase. One symptom to watch out for is a loss of their sense of time. You'll notice them repeatedly glancing at the clock or constantly asking what time it is.

Some patients start this process earlier than others. A strong indication that they are advancing into the next stage occurs when their sleep patterns become disrupted.

Since they can't remember what happened two minutes ago, it becomes arduous for them to estimate any time lapse. There are some patients that even become unable to distinguish day from night.

Keeping them in a simple routine helps them to maintain some perception of time. When they have their breakfast, lunch and dinner at the same time daily, they will at least have some sentience of what part of the day it is. A routine lifestyle will help them maintain their circadian or biological rhythm.

My father wore a wristwatch religiously, as if it was part of his physique. This did absolutely nothing for his time recognition, enhancing only his appearance. Why look at your wrist when you can ask the person next to you forty times, "What time is it?"

The human body adapts to what time it awakens every morning, sometimes to the point where an alarm clock is no longer necessary. But this is not the case with Alzheimer's patients!

It's well known that time passes by faster as we become older. In contrast, a seven-year-old may feel as if it takes an eternity between Christmases, but for an older adult it's, "Wow, the holidays are already here."

Once again, I despise saying that Alzheimer's patients revert to their childhood, but this is an accurate statement in more ways than one. If an Alzheimer's patient stood and watched a pot of water boil, it would become straight-out torture for them. Unfortunately, their attention span will grow shorter as the disease advances.

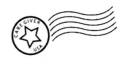

Dear Caregiver,

American writer Washington Irving, who was called "The Father of American Letters," said: "There is sacredness in tears. They are not the mark of weakness, but of power. They speak more eloquently than ten thousand tongues. They are messengers of overwhelming grief ... and unspeakable love."

This is such a beautiful and powerful statement.

GJL

Pain of Depression

(Loneliness, Depression, and Persistent Crying)

Despair is the first feeling that comes to mind; the hopelessness of caring for victims of Alzheimer's, knowing they are on a one-way street, heading toward their concluding address.

Next comes isolation—a constant cloudy overcast. It's not easily understood how one could feel alone while caring for a patient 24/7. But when treasured conversations dissolve, and you're barely recognized, trust me, loneliness creeps in surrounding you like a dense sea fog.

Depression is always strongest when the caregiver is overcome with fatigue. These are a few signs to watch for:

- Constant sadness
- Hopelessness
- Disruptive sleep patterns
- Fatigue
- Feeling worthless or guilty
- Significant weight change
- Loss of concentration
- Apathy

Many caregivers turn to alcohol and medications for escape, forgetting that this only adds weight to the burden of fatigue. Physical and mental exhaustion from substance abuse prevents the caregiver from ever catching up.

Sharing your feelings with a support group might do wonders. There are also several online chat rooms in which caregivers have an opportunity to vent. Keep in mind though, talking about stressors doesn't necessarily mend them. It's often necessary to go back to the origin of the problem.

If you're worried, remember, it's only natural. Try not to let it beat you up. Stay in touch with family and friends. Sometimes after a simple phone conversation, you'll feel a burden lift from your chest, at least long enough to catch your second breath. If necessary, talk with your physician. There's nothing to be ashamed of; you're doing a job most people wouldn't even attempt in the first place.

Understandably, depression is also widespread among those afflicted with Alzheimer's disease. In most cases, their downheartedness grows as their memory loss and the inability to live a normal life increases.

I've talked with many fellow caregivers who have told me that their loved ones go through a period of uncontrollable weeping, sometimes to the point where they are left almost breathless.

I often found my dad sitting at our kitchen table with tears in his eyes. This would happen during the early afternoon, a time of day when he really should have been at his best. During his brief moments of clarity he became acutely aware of what was happening to him and waves of sadness would sweep over him.

I witnessed how hard he struggled with his pride, trying desperately to hold himself together, especially in my presence. But it seemed that when my sister was with him, he would often drop his guard and occasionally cry for over an hour.

Persistent crying is, without doubt, a sign of depression and is an issue that should be brought immediately to the attending physician's attention.

Also, don't forget to attempt to divert their thoughts on to more pleasant memories from the past. Reminisce about something that has some kind of happy emotional attachment to them. This will be a much better strategy than to perpetually ask them, "What's wrong?" But unfortunately, with this disease, there comes a time when redirection will no longer do its job.

Try to decipher whether or not the tears are flowing from emotional or physical pain. Hopefully, this is something the physician will thoroughly investigate prior to treatment for major depression. Remember that it is well known that while someone is depressed they may also endure severe headaches along with other frequent body pains.

Antidepressant medications have been very effective in treating people suffering from Alzheimer's. As I've stated before, I truly believe that if their anxiety and depression are under control, they will manage a hundred times better throughout the course of the disease.

Do your best to maintain a realistic expectation of what your loved one can or cannot do. Expecting too much will only bring on additional frustration, possibly causing both of you to become more emotionally upset.

Please make sure you are not blaming yourself. Take comfort in knowing that these symptoms are generated from the disease itself. As the caregiver, actively anticipate these breakdowns taking place along the road of your journey.

It's always devastating to watch someone you care about cry incessantly, but keep in mind that hugs were invented to let someone know you love them without even saying a word.

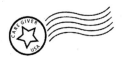

Dear Caregiver,

American philosopher and poet Ralph Waldo Emerson wrote: "It is one of the most beautiful compensations of life that no man can sincerely try to help another without helping himself."

You will find that after being a caregiver, you will have a different and better outlook on life.

GJL

Caregiver Stress

A fellow caregiver presented me with a leaflet about caregiver stress. Inside I found a cosmopolitan magazine-type questionnaire. I answered seven out of eight questions "yes" only to read at the bottom, "If you answered any of the above questions *yes*, you are probably experiencing *Caregiver Stress*." Just reading that presumptive evaluation was enough to make my blood pressure climb; myself, I didn't feel stressed out. Was I under pressure? "Yes, without a doubt."

I've always emphasized that all Alzheimer's patients react differently and I'm convinced this also falls true for caregivers. A large amount of tension comes from the actual caregiver feeling guilty, thinking that an adequate or acceptable job is not being performed. I offer here a truism: "There's no such thing as a perfect caregiver."

Take a moment to analyze your situation. Identify what you can reasonably expect to change or not change. Then concentrate on what is fixable and try not to let the rest overcome you. I know this is easier said than done.

Another risk for a caregiver is becoming physically exhausted. Keep a sharp eye out for signs of for the following:

· Irritability
· Loneliness
· Feeling overwhelmed
· Chronic headaches or body pains
· Weakness
· Dizziness
· Nausea or vomiting
· Weight change—up or down
· Heavy perspiration

When such physical symptoms occur, it's more than likely time to ask for help and train yourself to accept it.

Being a caregiver is an extremely arduous job. Therefore, it is especially important that you maintain your own personal health. One problem will most likely be that almost every spare second of your day is already consumed; so you begin cancelling your medical appointments. Also, the financial burden of caring for an Alzheimer's patient may result in no longer refilling much needed prescriptions for yourself!

Please try to remember that through all these difficulties, caring for your loved one does have its rewards. The fact that you're needed makes you feel worthy and helps you learn to appreciate life more fully. Ernest Hemingway advised, "To endure, one must laugh." You must keep your sense of humor and chuckle at the unbelievable things that are bound to happen.

Keep in mind, company employees covered by the Federal Family and Medical Leave Act may be able to take up to twelve weeks of "unpaid" leave per year to care for ailing relatives. You definitely don't need to lose your job with today's economy.

Make a habit of setting a certain amount of time aside for yourself each week. Spoil yourself, even if it's only for a couple of hours.

Dear Caregiver,

I love what Marcus Aurelius said on living, "The art of living is more like wrestling than dancing." Maybe he did his share of caregiving himself.

GJL

Last Stage Stress

You feel the tension building—crawling under your skin, believing you're failing at your everyday caregiver duties. All of the demands the world is making on you are steadily boiling to the point where you feel as though you'll erupt like Mount St. Helens.

These are normal signs of the stress a caregiver suffers while going through an Alzheimer's patient's last stage. You have to understand that, yes, these are indications of stress and depression, but it's natural and every caregiver is bound to endure them.

Spend time talking with someone who has gone through this—possibly via a local support group. For example, the thought of wishing the whole thing would be finished or pleading that it will come to a rapid and sudden end, will likely result in a *tsunami* of guilt within you. This is a common occurrence. You are not alone here; six out of ten adults will become a caregiver at some point in their lives and all must fight their way through the phenomenon.

The last stage of this disease is grueling. You will need help. In all reality, at least two people are required in order to successfully get through this ordeal. You will need more time-outs than ever. Take time to clear your head. I'm not trying to frighten you, but this ravaging mind-robbing villain erodes all of your loved ones' last strongholds.

My dad pointed at a photograph of me and told me that it was a picture of someone totally different—there wasn't even a close resemblance. I noticed that my father became extremely sensitive during the early part of this last stage, constantly apologizing and thanking me for the care he received. Even when he was not aware of who I was, he was still grateful for the affection I gave him.

Remember, you must have extra help and a prayer to get through this devastating finale.

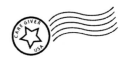

Dear Caregiver,

Lao Tzu, father of Taoism, once said: "Being deeply loved by someone gives you strength, while loving someone deeply gives you courage."

GJL

Stages of Alzheimer's

I've heard so many different theories regarding the number of different stages that can be experienced throughout the duration of Alzheimer's disease. Some experts have concluded that there are as many as fifteen different stages, but on the average I hear most declare that there are seven categories.

Personally, I believe it's best to break it down to only three stages: mild, moderate and severe.

The last thing the patient or caregiver needs to be worrying about is, are they now advancing into the eleventh or twelfth stage of the disease? Please relax and realize that these "stages" were only set up as general guidelines to keep caregivers and patients informed as to what to expect next.

First of all, the rate of the progression of Alzheimer's disease varies immensely. Not everyone will experience the same symptoms or advance at the same rate. Some will only live a short six years while others may survive up to twenty!

The following are some of the symptoms of the disease as broken down into three stages:

Mild Stage:

- Short-term memory loss.
- Difficulty with problem solving.
- Change in personality.
- Difficulty in expressing thoughts.
- Losing or misplacing things.

Moderate Stage:

- Increasingly poor judgment.
- Advanced confusion.
- Increased memory loss.
- Assistance needed for daily activities.
- Significant changes in personality and behavior.

Severe Stage:

- Losing the ability to communicate.
- Needs daily assistance with daily care.
- Loss of motor skills.

In a seven-stage arrangement, you can almost delete the first two stages since such minimal impairment is listed. The three-stage formula has less confusion which is something every caregiver needs.

The main reason I think it is important to know what stage your afflicted one is enduring is so that you, the caregiver, will have some kind of idea of what is coming next. This way you can make plans for the future without being too caught off guard.

Dear Caregiver,

You have to love this Russian Proverb on medicine: "Expensive medicines are always good, if not for the patient, at least for the druggist."

I have to say, there's a lot of truth in that statement.

GJL

Administering Drugs

One of the jobs that every caregiver will have to perform is the daily dispensing of medications. Dealing with all the new drugs in today's world, this task can become extremely confusing. In a twenty-four-hour period, a caregiver may have to administer medications as much as four or five times, possibly more.

This becomes a major battle when caring for Alzheimer's patients. They may argue that they already took their pills that morning.

Be sure to store their medication in a safe location; out of sight, out of mind. Leaving their pills in open view may have patients thinking that they haven't taken them and possibly digesting an extra dose. This could be most dangerous. For instance, they may be prescribed a blood thinner or some other kind of heart medication, the results could be devastating.

Caregivers also need to be cautious when dispensing over-the-counter medication. Consult with a pharmacist to make sure there will be no interactions with the prescribed drugs the patients are currently taking.

Also, if patients are diabetic, you need to watch all their medications' sugar content closely.

Trying to juggle the many caregiving duties all at once is a difficult act. I found it very helpful to set up all prescriptions in a weekly dispenser that has at least three compartments for each day. Not only was this less time consuming, but I could easily catch myself if I accidently missed distributing my father's medication at certain periods of the day. I believe filling this container should be left to only one person who knows the pill routine by heart and will notice right away if something is out of order. Then, if needed, another person can dispense directly from the prearranged container.

It is estimated that 60 percent of our elders have trouble swallowing their medications. When caring for Alzheimer's patients, you will learn that as the disease progresses, they will most likely have a chronic problem with swallowing, for this is one of the symptoms of the disease. This leads to most nurses and caregivers resorting to crushing their pills and mixing it into foods such as yogurt or puddings.

But be advised, crushing pills can lead to serious complications, including death!

Some pills often have a special coating that affects how the medicine is released into the body. Crushing them can disturb this complex system, discharging the medicine too fast, possibly causing an overdose. If this type of pill is prescribed to take once a day, what now could be happening is that all the medicine is released at once and the proper dosage is lacking throughout the rest of the day. Always talk to your pharmacist. In this circumstance, he or she may advise breaking the pill in half and administer the crushed dosage twice a day.

When you first start to notice that your loved one is having problems swallowing, speak with his or her attending physician. There may be alternatives to which form the medicine can be prescribed. It may also be available in liquid, patches, through inhalers, or even suppositories.

When available, the liquid form became a blessing toward the end of my father's life. I never even told him what I was about to do; I just asked him to open his mouth and then I would insert the medication gently along his gums; this made things nice and easy.

There are also precautions that should be taken for the person who is doing the crushing. It is always wise to use an actual pill crusher or at least place the pill inside of a ziplock bag before turning into granules. This way, you are not inhaling any of the dust (Be especially cautious if you're pregnant.)

Once again, speak with your doctor and pharmacist about your options. Figure out what works best for your loved one and yourself. I know from my past experience that the dispensing of my father's medications was a task that constantly weighed heavily on my mind while caring for him.

It may come to a point where you have to ask yourself if you are only treating the disease and no longer the patient. Have a discussion with the patient's physician. See if he or she still need be on everything currently prescribed. It may be possible that they have passed the point where these medications are doing any good.

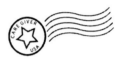

Dear Caregiver,

An unknown author wrote: "The happiest of people don't necessarily have the best of everything; they just make the most of everything they have."

GJL

Alcohol and Alzheimer's

I have often been asked for advice and/or my opinion on whether those suffering from Alzheimer's should be allowed to consume alcohol. Once again, I have no medical degree but from my personal experience, my answer is always emphatically "No!"

First of all, you must take into consideration the medications often prescribed for these patients; they can be incredibly strong. For example, my dad was taking Nemenda for nearly a year and a half. This medication threw off his equilibrium to the point where I was constantly worrying about him falling. Just the thought of having added alcohol to his system would have been insane.

The few other powerful drugs available for treating Alzheimer's: Exelon, Aricept and Axona are just as potent. Mixing alcohol with them can cause nausea, vomiting, headaches, drowsiness, fainting, internal bleeding and loss of coordination.

Secondly, even if your loved one is not currently taking any of these drugs, the consumption of alcohol will only increase his or her confusion, which is the exact opposite of what you will be trying to achieve.

I'm well aware of the fact that there are many people who have developed the habit of ending a long day of work by winding down and enjoying a drink, my father included. He loved to have a few glasses of wine in the evening, so naturally I found it necessary to dispose of all the liquor in the house, and then I kept it that way.

The first time the Hospice doctor came to the house, my father was sitting at the kitchen table with a wine glass in his hand. Dad, delighted to have a gentleman close to his age to sit and talk with, ordered me to pour the doc a glass of wine and told his new friend to pull up a chair and share a drink with him. The doctor, obviously stunned, stared at me. I quietly informed him that it was only cranberry juice. What they don't know won't hurt them. By serving Dad's juice in a wineglass or brandy snifter, helped him remain content, believing that he was still enjoying those distilled grapes from the past.

Although this worked well for my father, I'm sure many patients will put up a first-rate expostulation, demanding to have an alcoholic beverage in the same manner in which they are accustomed. I believe trying a bit of innocent deception is a tactic worth attempting. If beer is their beverage of choice, try switching to O'Doul's or some other brand of nonalcoholic ale.

Keep in mind that alcohol is a depressant. I don't have to tell anyone who has spent time around an Alzheimer's patient that, sadly, there's already enough depression brewing for everybody.

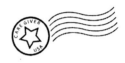

Dear Caregiver,

William Shakespeare, who certainly needs no introduction, wrote:"By divine instinct men's minds distrust danger."

Having been a male caregiver myself, I received many a soul-stirring direction about when things might go wrong. My advice is to listen to those inner feelings; they will guide you in the right direction.

GJL

Today's Male Caregivers

An estimated 40 percent of the caregivers in the United States are middle-aged men or older. It appears that these men are rolling up their sleeves, jumping in and getting their hands dirty. Whether caring for an elderly parent or an ill spouse, more and more are in it for the long haul, committing themselves to always "be there" for their loved one.

For generations, women have typically been the caregivers for any family members in need. This was often due to men being the primary breadwinners and women being at home and available. Times have certainly changed and since caregiving duties can be divided according to work schedules and not gender, my advice is, communicate with any employers involved, explaining about the circumstances and what to anticipate in the near future. Attempt to work out a plan that will satisfy everyone involved (Retaining employment may not only be important because of financial matters, but also medical insurance coverage and maybe even personal self-satisfaction.)

According to research, male caregivers are more likely to hold their emotions inside, creating more stress by not opening up and talking about their feelings. Men also refrain from asking for help until it is far too late—kind of like, never asking for directions till they become completely lost on a road trip.

As a male and my father's caregiver for ten years, I always tried not to show any weakness. I knew my father was always counting on me and I never wanted to disappoint him. I felt as if my manhood was at stake. The bottom line here is that not everyone can do this job. Don't be ashamed if you can't handle it. This might haunt you for the rest of your life and I'm sure that is not what your loved one would have wanted for you. If you cannot deal with it, find someone who can and remain a supportive kinsman in his or her life.

Focus on the positive aspects of caregiving. I believe what kept me going the most was the companionship I shared with my dad. This may sound peculiar considering that throughout the last years of his life, he hardly recognized who I was, but, I will never regret the years that I spent with him. They just may have been the most exceptional time of my life.

So to my fellow male caregivers, these are the things you need to concentrate on—staying healthy, learning to ask for assistance, keeping some sort of social life, and most of all maintaining a positive attitude.

As the Marines constantly cheer "Semper Fi," meaning "Always Faithful."

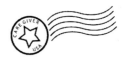

Dear Caregiver,

It is difficult to care for a loved one when you're far away. Keep in mind the following quote written by an unknown author, and it just might help you get a few more miles down the road: "Distance means so little when someone means so much."

GJL

Long–Distance Caregiving

(Family Spirit, Family Meetings and Hospice)

If you're attempting to care for ailing parents or relatives from across county and/or state lines, you are not alone. In the United States alone, approximately seven million long-distance caregivers are doing the same.

Worrying about loved ones from so far away is a difficult and nerve-wracking problem; are they eating sufficiently, taking their medications as prescribed or are they merely just safe?

Today's economy makes matters even worse. Your usual two-or-three trips per year to check on loved ones may be cutback to just one, due to financial constraints. If this is the case, plan carefully and in advance to assure that you make the most of your visits.

Prearrange an appointment with the patient's doctor so you can be present during the examination. Introduce yourself and explain the situation to the physician. Leave your contact information with the doctor and request that you be advised of any changes. Have a complete list of medications and dosages to take home with you. Always keep it updated. Even if you're not the person administering the drugs, you'll never know when this information might be essential.

Acquaint yourself with their neighbors and friends. Ask if they will periodically check on them; this way you'll have a reliable inside source. Leave several contact numbers if possible. Remember, you cannot rely on what you hear while talking to your afflicted loved one over the phone. They might sound absolutely fine, hang up and have no recollection of even talking to you. You simply cannot have any confidence in these conversations.

When you're visiting their home, see if there is edible food in the refrigerator. Also check for piles of unopened mail to see if bills are being paid promptly. Search out any safety issues. You might need to spend time making repairs or perhaps adding safety features such as support bars in the bathroom. Be sure to discard all throw rugs.

Just by inspecting the bathroom, you might be able to tell if they are practicing good personal hygiene without asking any embarrassing questions.

Here's a big one; make certain whether or not it's time to have their driving privileges revoked.

Now, if there's another family member performing the task of the primary caregiver, make sure that person receives some respite when the opportunity arises.

Caregivers that are most successful are the ones that receive support and love from family members and friends. If at all possible, don't let them run this campaign alone. They will only wear themselves out.

Communication will always be one of your best assets. It's important that family members hear what is constantly going on, for the caregiver's well-being and the sake of your loved one.

If you are the primary caregiver, ask a family member or close trusted friend to keep a caregiving notebook. Have them write down anything they feel is important from the regular conversations you are having. These notes should also include the date of birth, Social Security number, Medicare or Medicaid and insurance information, along with a list of physicians and medications.

Find someone that you can depend on to hold on to this crucial data in case something happens to you. The more support you have, even if it's just a pat on the back, the better. This will make each day that much easier to get through.

You will probably be able to handle most everything during the beginning stages of the disease. But down the road, when you come to the later stage, you're going to need some assistance. The earlier you learn to accept this, the better. You will be pleasantly surprised as I was that your "family" expands to include nurses, nurses' aides and many others who were formerly strangers to you.

At one point my dad's doctor tried to advise me to have him become a hospice patient. At first I was opposed to this idea and discarded it for an entire year before finally submitting. I believe the reason I most likely put this off was the mere fact that in my mind, I was relating the word *Hospice* with death, which is far from true. I wasn't ready to accept that we were actually nearing that point. Well, I was wrong, and if I had to do it again, I would have had Hospice helping me with my dad when the doctor first suggested it.

What I have learned is that Hospice is about comfort, not dying. When I finally did have them involved with my dad's care, he lived almost six months to the date he was signed up. But I could have used some vital help way before that. I will say that having Hospice there was nothing short of a blessing. And yes, there were a few members on the staff that within that short period of time almost felt as if they were family.

One of the most essential parts of caregiving is developing a plan with people you can count on.

Don't let this barbarous disease tear your family apart; if anything, it should bring your family closer together.

Remember that old saying "When the going gets tough, the tough get going." Well, if the family sticks together, everything will become easier and you'll be able to enjoy the time you have left with loved ones.

Everyone needs to understand that their independent living is coming to a halt, probably faster than anyone perceives.

Each time a long-distance caregiver takes a trip to visit, they will most likely have to stay a little longer. This is why family planning should be made a priority from the earliest possible moment after the diagnosis.

If several family members are involved, have a telephone date that involves conference calling. Schedule these group discussions ahead of time, for instance, the last Sunday evening of each month.

Canvass the patients' local churches, temples and community groups to see if meal delivery is an option. Also, do they provide transportation to and from appointments? If they don't, they'll most likely enlighten you on who does.

The Caregiver

People know that someday they may need a helping hand
and helping others help to make a person understand.
Two words come together explaining far and wide,
There is a special person, who will stand by your side.
You'll find that in a "Caregiver," Love is always in their heart
their thoughtful care and guidance gives each day its start.
Meeting needs of loved ones, helping them along the way,
repays the deeds they did for you each and every day.
A gentle touch a helping hand, the peace that's in a smile
they know how to comfort you, they go that extra mile.
It's not for fame or glory that they put your mind to ease
It's showing love to loved ones with Alzheimer's disease.
You'll find that there is peace and love until the end of
time being there for someone, helps to makes your spirit climb.

Esther Marie Latz

Hiring a Caregiver

(Care Managers and Outside Caregivers)

When reaching the age that some have oddly called "*the golden years,*" intrusive physical or mental health issues may initiate a time when it is no longer safe for the elderly to be left alone for short or long periods.

Hiring a caregiver may become necessary. This can prove to be incredibly difficult and even scary. The average person is used to living a private life and the thought of inviting perfect strangers into his or her home might seem quite distasteful. But in truth, it's actually a courageous and intelligent act.

Here is a short list of questions you should ask during the initial interview: Why have you chosen caregiving as a profession? Do you have a heart for this type of work or is it just a job? How much experience do you have in caregiving? What professional licenses do you possess (CNA, LPN, RN, or social worker)? Can you provide any health-care related references? Do you carry any liability insurance or are you bonded? Will this be your only case? Will you authorize a general background check? If lifting of patients is involved, are you healthy and strong enough to do so safely?

When it comes to the caregiver being paid, and if this is coming out of your own pocket, speak with an attorney and/or accountant to make sure all payroll taxes are being handled correctly. Just this subject alone may be reason enough to go through an agency, although there are countless success stories of the hiring of individuals on a private basis. They often come to be loved, accepted, and trusted as one of the family.

If this venture is to be a successful one, keep in mind that all parties need to be happy. Requiring timely arrival for the shift and being certain the caregiver is ready both physically and emotionally to "take over" is essential. When appropriate, be sure the caregiver has eye contact with and even a gentle touch for their patients. Next, get off on the right foot by providing an update on the patients' history since the caregiver was last there. Any skin tears? Bowel movements? Eating problems? Falls? Behavior changes? Yes, this new person in your home is working for you now, but is also an individual with a life and feelings of his or her own. If you can leave them a favorite soda or juice, anything to make them feel appreciated, it may do wonders in bringing your relationship into a feeling of teamwork.

If possible, having family and friends pitch in could also be a big help as well. Leave phone numbers of these important people with the caregiver.

Everyone desires independence. But the reality is, sometimes the simplest things in life that you or a loved one always attended to without the need of any assistance, such as bathing, dressing, shopping, housecleaning or driving may now have become difficult or near impossible tasks.

The heart of the matter is: *your loved one needs help.* And if there is no one to depend on and they want to remain living in their own home, you will eventually need the assistance of an outside caregiver. If they wait too long to put this into place, institutional care may not be far off.

A family crisis is what usually prompts the initial thought of bringing in a care manager. A son or daughter realizes that a parent's dementia or other health problem has reached a point to where he or she shouldn't be left unattended.

Looking back at the circumstances I went through with my dad, I cannot think of a time when I actually needed the assistance of a care manager; but that's because I was available to him 24/7. However, having a care manager would be an ideal situation for anyone attempting to be a long-distance caregiver. This person could be nothing less than a priceless team player.

This is going to be an extra expense, but once you overcome the original cost and a plan has been drafted and put into place, the relief you feel from not having to constantly worry about loved ones will make the money spent well worth it. Finally, you will have someone to confer with and give you an update regarding the latest in their life. That alone will be very comforting.

Your care manager may not be the one providing hands-on care, but they will coordinate and supervise the ones that are.

A care manager must be able to do a comprehensive assessment and reassessment, develop a care plan, and implement the monitoring of quality evaluations.

One concern I would have is how many cases the care manager is currently handling; for instance, if they have twenty active cases that should raise a red flag. Also, be sure to ask for references. Hiring this person and taking their advice is part of providing for the welfare of your loved ones.

Always remember: you have the final say. Never push aside those intuitive inner feelings; someone still needs to watch the watchman.

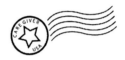

Dear Caregiver,

A three=time Pulitzer winner Carl Sandburg wrote:"Valor is a gift. Those having it never know for sure whether they have it until the test comes."

As a caregiver, you will find these words to be ever so true.

GJL

Accepting an Outside Caregiver

One of the most common dilemmas involved in caregiving is getting aging parents or friends to admit when they need help. Just the thought of their independence being in question is terrifying and humiliating to them.

More than half of seniors will refrain from ever asking for help, even from one of their own adult children or siblings. This attempt of self-preservation is usually the cause of many family spats, escalating into some intense altercations that go way beyond the simple silent treatment.

And unfortunately, those suffering from Alzheimer's or dementia can become experts at maintaining the appearance that all is well during the earlier stages of the disease, some to the point where they become a danger to themselves.

Seniors who survived the Great Depression and World War II eras are passionately private people and often quite stoic. They come from a proud upbringing and will fight for every last bit of independence they have.

Women from this generation took pride in being homemakers and actually being the caregiver for their families. Men were known as breadwinners. This makes it a lot more difficult for them to accept benevolent assistance from anybody, all the way up to when it's time to start to climb Jacob's ladder.

In those days, it was just a given fact of life that if Grandma or Grandpa got ill, they would live with one of their children, grandchildren or, in some instances, a cousin or other relative. The phenomenon of "the nursing home" was a concept that seems to have snuck in during postwar America. It appears that families were so busy chasing The American Dream during the 1950's, 1960's, and so on that institutionalizing ill relatives became the norm.

Now, the real problem lies with trying to get them to accept having a stranger in their home to help them. Most will put up a battle even having their own daughter or son running their household.

It's best to try to ease them into this new lifestyle gradually. Tell them that you wish only to try this new caregiver for an hour or two and then gradually increase the length of time they spend together. It's important that your loved one still feels that they still have some control. Assure them that if it doesn't work, you'll find someone else.

You will have to hear a lot of accusations of how the "intruders" are stealing from them, talking behind their back, etc. My dad would become extremely verbally abusive at times. But if the caregivers are professionals, they should be able to brush those defamations off their capable shoulders.

Hopefully, you can help your loved one to gradually adapt. Eventually, he or she might actually look forward to the caregiver's visits.

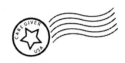

Dear Caregiver,

British poet and philosopher Samuel Coleridge wrote: "I have often thought what a melancholy world this would be without children, and what an inhuman world without the aged."

GJL

A Child's Role in Alzheimer's Care

A caregiver's age can vary from twelve-year-old to someone in their nineties. Many families welcome parents and grandparents with Alzheimer's into their home to care for them and keep them safe.

There will be times, though, when a parent might need to ask his or her teenage son or daughter to watch the memory-impaired grandparent while the parent is out running errands or just going out for the evening. If you have a responsible teen, by all means, go out as a couple and try to maintain the romance in your relationship. The stress of caregiving is notorious for ripping families apart.

Explain to all of your children exactly what's going on with their grandparent. Young people are quite keen on what is happening around them. Withholding information in an attempt to shield them from confusion or pain will ultimately make the situation worse. Assure them that this disease is not contagious.

Express that there will be plenty of unfamiliar behavior and changes coming from the grandparent and that they shouldn't be alarmed.

Children tend to be flexible and will usually bounce back quickly from the strong emotions that will constantly be surrounding them while living with an Alzheimer's patient.

Prepare them ahead of time that the grandparents with Alzheimer's will eventually forget their names and even who they are. They'll most likely shout at the kids for making too much noise or running in the house. My father had absolutely no recognition of any of his grandchildren or great-grandchildren during the last few years of his life.

Once again, point out that the patient is not to blame for his or her odd behavior; it is a direct result of the advancement of the disease.

There are some children who relate well to memory-impaired loved ones and develop a special relationship with them. You may wish to enlist their help with simple caregiving chores to help care for their grandparents.

What you might have to be concerned with is those few times when kids can be mean. Teasing or ridiculing the patient will cause a mountain of confusion. It's sad to say, but there could be times when they may need to be protected from their own grandchildren.

If this is the case, have another heart-to-heart talk with them. Youngsters may be acting out from feeling cheated that their parents are spending quality time with the one they're caring for rather than with them.

It's heartbreaking enough for an adult to witness what happens to a loved one dying from Alzheimer's;

just imagine how devastating it is for a grandchild. When you tell a young child that Grandpa Joe isn't crazy, he's dying from a fatal disease, it is difficult for any kid to understand. I firmly believe it's best to prepare them now instead of trying to explain death, when everybody is an emotional wreck. Honesty works best with children.

You may want to arrange a meeting with the children's school. Talk to their teachers and counselors explaining the circumstances at home. Their behavior might become noticeably different when they are away attending class.

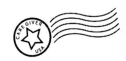

Dear Caregiver,

Fred Allen, old=time radio show host said:"If the grass is greener in the other fellow's yard, let him worry about cutting it."

The way I look at it is, don't let anyone distract you from your main objective; keeping your loved one safe and content.

GJL

The Difference between Alzheimer's and Dementia

After spending much time conferring with the general public, I have come to the conclusion that a large percentage of people have a hard time distinguishing the difference between Alzheimer's and dementia.

Recently, I was thrilled to read an article that simply explained that, "Dementia is a symptom, and Alzheimer's is the cause of the symptom. A good analogy to the term 'dementia' is 'fever.' Fever refers to an elevated temperature, indicating that the person is sick, but it does not touch on any information on what is causing the sickness." So basically what it's saying is that dementia is not the disease, it is one of the symptoms of the disease.

There are many causes of dementia and some are reversible. But unfortunately, 70-80 percent of all cases occur from Alzheimer's which is not reversible. In fact, it is fatal!

The word "dementia" has come to replace many old terms such as senility, having senior moments or experiencing a second childhood. And it is important to know that dementia is not necessarily a normal part of aging. If it does present itself, persons showing signs should be checked out thoroughly. The significance of a correct diagnosis could make all the difference in putting them on the right track and possibly curing the problem.

Now that we have differentiated that dementia is a symptom, what are the characteristics to look for? Well, the most prominent one is the loss of memory, which leads into the decline of other cognitive skills such as language, attention span, decision-making and motor skills functions.

Fighting for the cause against Alzheimer's includes educating the public to be aware of all the disabilities involved with the disease. This also means educating physicians. Over the past several years, many doctors have seemed to become at ease with the inclination of diagnosing the patient with Alzheimer's a little too quickly when, in fact, it may be a form of dementia that could be reversible.

So remember this, when dealing with Alzheimer's or dementia, beginning with a proper diagnosis is essential so that the patient can immediately be pre-scribed the correct treatment or therapy and the family can plan ahead from this point and get started on the right foot.

Our Friend Who Was and Is

A Shadow on the sun
his mind and heart came to us
our lives were joined

He said to us,
The sun is just a cooking egg
in the spiral pan of now.
We are in the white of it,
specks of pepper giving grief to the void,
Succeeding against odds to keep the taste of time—

We saw him striding
just in the fading music of the dusk
one foot on the curb, one in the street,
to feel in the moment's suspended doubling
to face the unusual

This forms a certain cadence—
the cadence of a street in light and shadow,
where life and death may have another name.
There he might run his fingers through his thoughts,
while the world blows his soul toward a picture—
The triptych mystery in our own momentary flame

A shadow on the moon
his heart and mind stay with us
though he is gone

Peter Hanen

Early–Onset Alzheimer's

Although symptoms of Alzheimer's usually begin to appear in people that are in their late sixties, there are an estimated two hundred thousand people under the age of sixty-five who have become afflicted with the disease. This is known as early-onset Alzheimer's and averages about 5 percent of those diagnosed. Studies show that there are cases of patients in their thirties and forties, but this is extremely rare.

The genetic path of inheritance is much greater in early-onset Alzheimer's. Those that have a parent or grandparent who developed the disease at a younger age have a higher risk of developing it themselves.

Many believe that early-onset Alzheimer's progresses at a faster rate. Although there is no hard evidence of this, I believe it to be true.

When this disease invades so early in life, a number of problems quickly unfold. These newly stricken patients may still be caring for a parent who is battling the same illness. Meanwhile, they may also have their own children still living at home. Their family members, neighbors and co-workers might ridicule and berate these poor people, calling them straight-out lazy, when the fact of the matter is Alzheimer's has destroyed their motivation for life.

Commonly, patients experience heavy bouts of depression and frustration. Often, marital problems develop from being misunderstood and undiagnosed.

According to the experts, 80 percent of these patients will lose their employment and their corresponding income.

Alzheimer's is devastating at any age, but it seems to be so much more unfair when it strikes at a younger age.

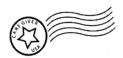

Dear Caregiver,

Rosalynn Carter was asked what her husband had that President Gerald Ford did not, her response was: "He has me!"

The fact that your loved one has you standing by their side is the best thing in their world.

GJL

Sex and Alzheimer's

(Disrobing, Fowl Language and Sexual Conduct)

Summoning the courage to ask a doctor (or anyone else for that matter), discomforting questions about Alzheimer's patients' sexual activity is a universal problem. Caregivers must understand that this conduct could be another fallout of the disease.

Disinhibition is a term in psychology, meaning "a lack of restraint including a disregard for social conventions." In other words, those suffering from cognitive impairment such as Alzheimer's, or other forms of dementia, may have shortcomings in areas of normal, social restraint.

For instance, they may begin to form a habit of disrobing in public or in front of anybody at home, including children. This may become an extremely embarrassing situation and is, of course, inappropriate behavior.

Try to discover what could be causing this poor deportment by analyzing the situation. Could something else be initiating this conduct? In many cases, there may be something environmental that's triggering it.

People with Alzheimer's may suddenly begin undressing simply because they are not comfortable. They could be feeling too hot or their clothes may be causing them to itch. Fortunately, there is the option of buying clothes designed specifically for Alzheimer's patients. Simply go online and Google the words "Alzheimer's clothing" and such items will pop-up. One such is a jumpsuit particularly designed with anti-disrobing features, including long zippers down the back complete with a dome closure behind the neck, so that the wearer can't get to the zipper head. But be aware that this change will now bring on the need of extra assistance in undressing for bathroom use, etc.

I found that the looser the clothes, the better my father accepted them. He absolutely refused to wear anything that even resembled a taut fit. As I said before, I couldn't even persuade him to wear socks for the last two years of his life. It was a good thing we lived in a usually warm Florida climate.

If you should find yourselves in a public place and they should begin to disrobe, try not to panic; first try redirection, attempt to turn their thoughts on to anything else besides their clothing. Also get yourself into the habit of bringing along extra clothing. Simply having them put on a fresh shirt may solve the problem.

As I have stated in earlier writings, redirection works best when you can actually hand them something they can touch, taste or smell. For example, if you're in a restaurant, try handing them a couple of pieces of silverware and ask them which one they like better or have them taste something and ask their gourmet opinion of the flavor.

At all cost, avoid becoming angry or embarrassing them. Remain composed, maybe finding somewhere private for them to sit quietly for a while. A crowd or unfamiliar faces could be the culprit, causing them to have a bout of anxiety.

Another example of inappropriate behavior you may encounter is obscene language. Even someone who rarely swore in public before may now be throwing out words that could make a trucker blush. If they become foul mouthed or verbally abusive, you may have to sit down and explain to adults and children alike who are within hearing range that it is the disease causing this poor behavior and that normally your loved one has always refrained from this kind of demeanor.

As far as dealing one-on-one, gently remind them that this behavior is unfitting.

If you're in a public place and you cannot divert their attention on to something else, it may be better to excuse yourselves and head back home where they will once again feel safe and secure.

When it comes to the subject of sexuality, disheartening changes in people with Alzheimer's will most likely bring about unwelcome behaviors. Patients may also experience an increase or decrease in their sex drive.

With so many spouses performing the role of caregivers, the patients may display rages of jealousy and might break into verbal or physical combativeness from not recognizing their partner. Sexual advances toward strangers usually occur due to the belief that a stranger is their companion.

A lack of attention span on the part of the patient might leave the partners without dementia disappointed or feeling unsatisfied during and after the union of sex. Such problems usually occur during the early to moderate stages of the disease. Sexual intercourse later becomes improbable due to the patients' general decline in physical stamina.

Sexual activity is a significant way for couples to maintain their love and affection. Having this taken away can be devastating. There are still many people who have a hard time accepting that senior citizens can be sexually active. But sympathy plays a pronounced role—bringing them emotionally closer, enhancing a sense of commitment.

The crumbling memory of an Alzheimer's patient can rip the heart of a caregiver right out. Thus, it becomes hard for one to maintain an interest in sex after caring for a loved one suffering from dementia all day. When a caregiver is mentally and physically exhausted, usually the thought of sex just flies right out the window.

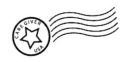

Dear Caregiver,

A doctor kept asking an Alzheimer's patient questions to check his cognition, "Do you ever hear voices without knowing who or where the voice is coming from?"

"Well, now that you mention it, I do," the patient told the doctor.

"When does this usually happen?"

"Usually when I answer the phone."

Being a caregiver, it won't take you long to see the dilemma of telephones and Alzheimer's.

GJL

Telephones and Alzheimer's

Commencing from my dad's earliest onset of Alzheimer's, it became obvious that answering the telephone was going to become an issue.

Back then, my father was still sitting behind the front counter of our bookstore. If he managed to grab the phone before I got to it, I would witness a blank stare evolve across his face. Sometimes he stayed completely voiceless as he held the receiver to his ear, then slowly he placed it back on its base. When I asked him who had just called, he would just nonchalantly respond, "Heck if I know." I realized we wouldn't be in business for very long if this continued.

I purchased a wireless headset and removed the telephone from behind the counter. This prompted my father into asking me straight-out, "So, I guess you don't want me answering the phone anymore?" My heart sank deep into my chest as I told him "No, I think it would be best if I cared for all business calls from now on."

Another problem was the phone in our store also rang in our house. I would be talking with a customer when all of a sudden my father would be putting his two cents worth in from our kitchen. Asking him to please hang up was pointless. Eventually, I shut off all the ringers on the phones near him in the house until our bill for long distance started having randomly dialed international calls. Finally this left me with absolutely no choice but to remove all phones in our house, except for one which stayed in my sleeping quarters.

More than one fellow caregiver has told me that their patient formed a habit of dialing 911 just to have a conversation with someone.

Expecting them to write messages down is just wishful thinking. This is where caller ID is useful because at least you can look back and see who called. Call forwarding also became handy; at times I would have all our calls transferred to my cell phone.

I'm just warning you now that as the Alzheimer's advances, your telephone will, without a doubt, become a dilemma. Planning and anticipating changes will ease some of the inevitable hardships and hurt feeling that lie ahead.

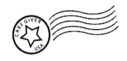

Dear Caregiver,

Maria Edgeworth was one of the first realist writers in children literature. She once wrote: "If we take care of the moments, the years will take care of themselves."

I found that if you worry about the smaller problems first, the larger ones seem to mend themselves.

GJL

Television and Alzheimer's

For many decades, medical researchers have spent both time and money exploring every avenue available in an attempt to find a cure for Alzheimer's. As this study continues, so does the courageous and yet ponderous undertaking by caregivers to navigate the daily maze of their loved ones' disorders.

As I've written many times in the past, "every patient responds differently," so just accept that trial and error will be a large part of figuring out what avocations help calm and subdue the confusion that abides within these poor souls.

Memory exercises and cognitive workouts are essential. I believe in that old saying "use it or lose it," so do your best to keep your loved ones' minds and hands occupied. This practice will benefit both patients and the caregivers by creating a few moments of peace.

One tool that I used, which is right at the fingertips of most people, is the television. Up until the last stage of my father's battle with this disease, I kept our television tuned on the Game Show Channel during the day. It didn't matter how old the reruns were (they could be giving away the grand prize of a 1984 Chevy), it made no difference to him. As long as a constant assortment of questions flowed through the air, his mind was kept active, searching for answers.

I recall him sitting at our kitchen table playing solitaire, with "Jeopardy" pulsating in the background, when suddenly I would hear him shout out what he believed to be the answer! Whether he was right or wrong isn't the point. The fact that he was stimulating a few brain cells is what matters.

In today's world, the ever-present living room box can easily be hooked up to a Wii game console. Throughout nursing homes and physical therapy centers across the nation, the Wii device is being used for physical and mental fitness along with instigating social interaction.

After our dinner hour, my father did very well watching baseball. We rarely missed a Tampa Bay Rays game. These sporting events had conveniently taken the place of the intense mystery shows he so much used to love. The "who done its" had simply become too much for him to manage. At least with televised baseball, there was always a perpetual scoreboard banner across the top of the screen.

(I will say that it's just not the same watching the games without him anymore. But I'm sure, he's still yelling at the players from his newly acquired, grand upper-deck seats.) The *Lawrence Welk Show* was another venue which worked quite well. He would casually sing along as if he wrote the lyrics himself.

Remember, it doesn't necessarily have to be the idiot box sounding off, a radio may be just as effective, as I said earlier, "trial and error." You just have to continue to explore different avenues and find what suits your situation best.

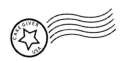

Dear Caregiver,

J. R. R. Tolkien, author of the fantasy epic "Lord of the Rings" wrote: "Remember what Bilbo used to say: 'It's a dangerous business, Frodo, going out your door. You step onto the road, and if you don't keep your feet, there's no knowing where you might be swept off to.'"

Traveling with an Alzheimer's patient is something that Bilbo would tell you should be deeply thought out.

GJL

Traveling Woes

(Vacations and Group Gatherings)

Occasionally, family members will understandably want to travel with a loved one who has advanced into the moderate stage of Alzheimer's. I have learned, however, that such travel can do more harm than good. If you must travel, try to do most of it during the earliest stage of the disease.

On one such journey, I saw my dad stare at me with an expression of total fear, cloaked in panic when he suddenly became clueless as to where he was or how he got there.

While on a trip to visit relatives in Canada, my dad literally lifted my ponderous body off the motel bed by my shirt collar at 3:00 a.m. Quite honestly, I would never have believed him to have that much strength left in his diminishing body. Screaming, he demanded to know where he was.

Although my ulterior motive had been to take my father for a final visit to see his beloved family members while he still knew who they were, I realized then I had paved a road to hell with good intentions. I had violated everything I'd preached! I had selfishly put miles between Dad and his everyday refuge.

At home, my father would spend hours with a deck of cards spread out in front of him, clinging to them as a safety net. I inadvertently stole this security blanket. So the next morning, I purchased a one-dollar deck of cards to help usher him back into his safety zone. Now, if counting numbers and matching red and black suites gave him security, he could play all the *solitaire* in the world!

If it becomes necessary to include your loved one with you along on a trip, be sure you bring something that he or she is familiar with:

- Crossword puzzles
- Jigsaw puzzles
- Checkers
- Photo albums
- Crafts

Anything they enjoy at home.

This will help keep both of you sane. Pushing something new on them when they are already out of sync will only create more chaos. If your loved one likes to knit, let him or her knit a scarf half a mile long. As said earlier, "There is something about repetition that produces a calming effect."

Many people have asked my opinion as to whether to take a person with Alzheimer's on a cruise or to a wedding. I've often heard horror stories from those who opted to do so, saying that everything that could have gone wrong, did. Then, after they finally returned home, it took days if not weeks for the patient to recover from being away from his or her accustomed environment.

Of course, there may be times when you simply have no choice and must take them along with you. Otherwise, you must look at the big picture and try to keep your loved one in a routine run-of-the-mill lifestyle. Thus, you can avoid years of apprehension and gain many days of them knowing exactly who you are.

Attending group gatherings, eating out at restaurants, and going on shopping trips are overwhelming for your Alzheimer's victim. If this insecure person panics when becoming lost in his or her own home, just imagine what fear your loved one will have to endure if lost in an unfamiliar location.

Providing a loving and safe home is the best thing you can do.

A Christmas View

Blinking lights in pine and fir trees;
lights of Christmas hues, enchant me.
Magic … really!

White and blue in rhythm blinking,
glimmer, shine, while chimes are tinkling.
Nog, for drinking.

Green of Christmas, lush as meadow;
red of ribbon, warm as heart glow
tie the love bow.

Blinking lights in colors, varied.
Man and Christ–child, Christmas married.
This I see!

Valerie Esker

An Alzheimer's Holiday

An overwhelming sense of loneliness often permeates Alzheimer's caregivers, especially during the holiday season. This can be caused by their social world collapsing around them and the feeling of being trapped in a domain of solitude.

This is a sensation that most people cannot grasp if they have never experienced the tribulations of serving as a primary caregiver. An outsider's mind can't understand how a caregiver could feel such a heavy weight of aloneness, when in reality they are never by themselves, always caring for someone 24/7.

If you are planning on taking on this difficult and noble job be prepared for vast changes. Running to the grocery store, visiting friends or just going for a drive may no longer be an option since you won't be able to leave your loved one alone, not even for a single minute. This all starts boiling together and you will likely experience the sensation of being isolated.

Unfortunately, these emotions may become more intense during the holiday season. This time of year is known for bringing on stronger bouts of depression. Your friends from the past are out celebrating the holiday festivals, Christmas parties or other family traditions. Your plans may be disrupted because simple family rituals have taken your Alzheimer's patient out of his or her daily routine. Like everybody else, the caregiver has extra errands to run in what feels like a shorter period of time—typical holiday madness.

Rather than dwell on the downside of things, here are certain steps you can take so that you and your loved one can enjoy the holidays.

First, try to hold the family celebration in a familiar environment. Taking patients to another family member's dwelling could prove too confusing for them. This could devastate everyone's holiday. I suggest celebrating quietly in the comfort of the beloved patient's own home.

Second, make sure to tone down the decorations. Blinking lights and large holiday displays will overwhelm any tranquility loved ones may achieve.

Third, once guests have arrived, refrain from having everyone visiting with their loved one all at once. Talk with the family ahead of time. Keep the traffic to a minimum. Trying to recognize too many faces at once or the sounds of multiple voices all talking at the same time will become extremely upsetting. If possible, limit gatherings to the daytime hours. Visiting at night when mental confusion is much more pronounced makes absolutely no sense.

Fourth, keep your patient's food choices to a minimum. There's enough turbulence going on already. The fewer decisions they have to make, the better.

A few Christmases ago, I thought my father would enjoy helping wrap presents. This proved to be a very painful and time-consuming mistake. Frustration and anxiety overwhelmed him as he was unable to remember whose gift he had just wrapped only to have him rip the packages back open, throwing him into a world of confusion.

Let them try to help with whatever task you believe they can still handle. You need to be calm and follow your instincts.

Holidays bring extra stress for everyone, but don't wear yourself down too thin. If you need assistance with the extra chores, don't be afraid to ask for help from a family member or friend.

The main thing is try to relax and enjoy the season. Hopefully, everything will remain peaceful. You just have to do the best that you can.

I can't tell you how many fellow caregivers have contacted me recently, expressing how they receive more help from close friends than from their own family members. They are overwhelmed by the reluctance of their own kin opting to do nothing to help the loved one they're sacrificing everything for.

This is where I suggest you stand up a little taller and don't let your relatives destroy your holidays. In fact, give them a call and wish them the best. Don't let these people distract you from achieving your main goal, which is caring for the one who needs you the most.

Try to have a calm and relaxing holiday. After all, the number of seasons you have left to share with your precious loved one is becoming fewer by the very nature of the disease. Even if you celebrate the day, just the two of you, at least you're together. To my way of thinking, this is actually the most essential issue. Someday, you may look back and wish that you still felt all that loneliness all over again just to still have your loved one in your life.

Dear Caregiver,

An unknown author wrote: "The happiest of people don't necessarily have the best of everything; they just make the most of everything they have."

GJL

Art and Music Therapy for Alzheimer's

My father, stricken with Alzheimer's as he was, always amazed me with his ongoing ability to recall the lyrics of old songs. Music from the television or radio would often strike a happy chord for him and he would sing out the lyrics with gusto.

Dr. Oliver Sacks, Professor of Neurology and Psychiatry of Columbia University, wrote that he has worked in a hospital and several old-age homes where, although many patients had Alzheimer's or other dementia-related diseases, he still discovered that, "All of them, without exception, responded to music."

He believes these patients have some of their personal memories "embedded in amber," in a manner of speaking. Things such as music can draw out some of these locked whispers from the past.

There is a part of the brain called the "Parietal Lobe" which responds to creative activities like art and music. The visual stimulation of viewing something artistically created can promote communication. Somehow, as if the piece of art is speaking directly to them, thoughts begin to generate. They may not be completely accurate in describing what they're seeing, but if it enhances conversation, there is something positive here.

The Museum of Modern Art in New York was one of the first to start a project for people with Alzheimer's. They put together a small collection of art that is accessible to a group of patients one day a month. Together they view a sampling of, for instance, Frederic Remington's work and then a different artist the following month. By keeping the collection small, the event organizers keep the visitors from becoming overwhelmed. The curator then engages the group with questions such as, "What do you think of the colors?" or "What do you make of this image?" The reports have contained surprising depths of observation coming from the patients.

I believe this type of therapy is healthy for Alzheimer's patients to attend, unless the trip becomes too unsettling for them. Anything that promotes conversation or energizes the mind, helping to give a richer quality of life, is extremely encouraging.

My dad had a deep love for fine art throughout his life and became a certified art appraiser. He loved to show off a painting that he owned and tell the history of the artist, when the picture originated, etc. One day, about halfway through his battle with Alzheimer's, I heard a woman asking him what he knew about a certain oil painting he owned. He knew exactly what region the landscape was painted from, even the right era! But when it came to the artist, he struggled and then told her, "Barnes and Noble painted this." The woman stared at me quizzically. I just gave her a gentle nod as to say, "Please, just let him continue." He may have not remembered all the correct details, but the man loved to shoot the breeze about his paintings.

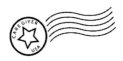

Dear Caregiver,

I don't think there is hardly anyone out there that hasn't read or heard of the comic strip "Peanuts" with its adorable character Snoopy, written by Charles Monroe Schulz. I believe one of his best named titles is "Happiness Is a Warm Puppy." Nothing could be more true.

GJL

Pet Therapy

Many caregivers are searching for natural health remedies these days. One treatment that I've discovered that takes the edge off the anxiety of Alzheimer's patients is a loveable pet.

When I was caring for my dad, there were times where he became saturated with confusion. I would simply place our cat named Kitty on his lap and casually tell him that Kitty was lonesome and in dire need of love and attention. Giving both his hands and his mind something to focus on, his panic seemed to evaporate as soon as the purring commenced.

A characteristic of Alzheimer's is the loss of ambition. Including a pet as part of their environment helps motivate these people with a sense of responsibility and purpose.

Many times I walked into our kitchen and found five bowls of milk on the floor; I never had to worry about our cat starving. Then my father would ask if I had fed the cat—repeatedly. But I soon learned our furry friend made my life easier.

Pet ownership has been associated with lowering blood triglyceride levels in the human body. This helps to increase activity and hopefully socialization.

Choosing a dog as a pet may help to encourage physical activities. It may even inspire the patient to play a bit or go for a walk, thus creating a sense of significance.

People with dementia are susceptible to loneliness and depression. Having a pet around will help break up the solitude that the forgetfulness creates.

Some pets even seem to be sensitive to their owners' needs and most of them enjoy attention. They don't get upset and walk away when hearing the same story over and over or hearing constant chatter that makes absolutely no sense. Perhaps they're better listeners or, at the very least, are not so judgmental.

The ideal pet is one that is calm and gentle, not hyperactive or loud. Select a new pet with great care. If your loved one has always been afraid of dogs, then obviously a dog is probably not the answer. Try an aquarium full of fish, a hamster, rabbit or even a bird; any pet that gives them a feeling of being needed.

Be watchful. You still have to observe the situation constantly. Innocently, they may overfeed the pet or attempt to walk the dog. These common occurrences just might leave you facing a spell of anxiety of your own.

If you find a pet that decreases a patient's anxiety and leaves him or her feeling calm, you've just accomplished an ample part of your goal.

Like any other type of intervention, this might not work for everyone. But I believe it's worth a try. If you have a friend or neighbor that owns a pet, ask them to bring their four-legged friend over for a visit. The results may indeed surprise you.

Little Things

It's just the little, homely things,
The unobtrusive, friendly things,
The "won't=you=let=me=help=you" things
That make our pathway light—
And it's just the jolly, joking things,
The "never=mind=the=trouble" things,
The "laugh=with=me, it's=funny" things
That make the world seem so bright.
For all the countless famous things
The wondrous, record=breaking things,
The "never=can=be=equaled" things
That all the papers cite
Aren't like the little human things,
The everyday=encountering things,
The "just=because=I=like=you" things
That make us happy quite.
So here's to all the simple things,
The dear "all=in=a=day's=work" things,
The "smile=and=face=your=troubles" things.
Trust God to put them right!
The "done=and=then=forgotten" things,
The "can't=you=see=I=love=you" things,
The hearty "I=am=with=you" things
That make life worth the fight.

Unknown Author

Informing Loved Ones That They Have Alzheimer's

Should we tell our loved ones that they are suffering from Alzheimer's? This is a dilemma all caregivers must face sooner or later.

First, let's consider what stage of the disease the patients are currently in. Obviously, the earlier the stage, the more they will be able to comprehend. But as the disease progresses, constantly informing them that they are showing symptoms may have little or no advantage.

Caregivers must use their own best-suited judgment pertaining to what they feel is correct in their own circumstance. There is no "how to" manual of rights and wrongs when it comes to dealing with this disease. Each patient responds differently.

At first, it's important for patients to have the opportunity to decide their own future care and the care of their dependents. Also, this may sound strange, but they will actually need some time to grieve about being given this dreadful diagnosis. This is a valid stage for them to walk through, which may help them to determine what choices are to be made in their own behalf.

You will always want to do what's best for them. Your initial reaction is naturally going to be to protect them from any further pain or distress. If you feel it's best not to awaken the memories of the diagnosis, make sure to tell other family members and friends so that you are all on the same page.

Now if you desire to go the other route, reminding them of the reason they are constantly confused, make sure it is done in a sensitive manner and then reassure them that you will always be there for them.

When discussing the matter, see how it goes at first. If you see that they are becoming upset, back off. Usually, the best time of day for them is going to be between 10:00 a.m. and 3:00 p.m.

Remember, this disease not only affects their ability to comprehend, it also affects their power to communicate. It's only fair that they should be given the opportunity to express concerns about what is happening to them.

I've always stated that denial is a symptom of the disease which seems to affect everyone involved. It's possible they might never actually accept there is something wrong with them. This is one situation where telling them may send them into a whirlwind of anxiety, doing more harm than good.

If you are the person who initially discovered strange behaviors or their acting out of character, then I would advise you to call their doctor, thus giving the physician a heads up that you feel there's something potentially wrong. But it is very common for patients to instruct their doctors not to tell anyone about their diagnosis. This is one of the problems with the disease which may cause a little bit of a dilemma for the physician. You may have a better chance of being brought in on the diagnosis if you're the one who initially raised the concern.

If you are certain that they should always be informed what is happening to them, be prepared to repeat yourself for many years to come. In the case of my father, I elected not to keep telling him. I felt there was no reason to bring up a subject matter that was followed by a wave of depression. Even if it lasted only for ten minutes, that's ten minutes too long.

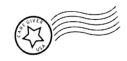

Dear Caregiver,

In the book "For Whom the Bell Tolls" Ernest Hemingway wrote: "If we win here, we win everywhere."
Finding a cure for this merciless disease of Alzheimer's would be a victory for the whole world.

GJL

Clinical Trials

If a cure for Alzheimer's is ever to be found, clinical studies are essential. Caregivers must carefully weigh the advantages and disadvantages of enrolling patients in such a study.

Participation will necessitate a serious commitment of time and effort on their part as well as the patients. There are details to consider and questions that need to be answered before making a decision.

First, caregivers must be able to accept the responsibility of transporting patients back and forth from the study's location as scheduled.

I believe one of the major drawbacks is the stripping of loved ones away from their daily routine. I truly learned from caring for my father for so many years how damaging this becomes and how important it is to keep an Alzheimer's patient in a run-of-the-mill lifestyle.

If you have faith that you, as a caregiver, can handle the extra stress—by all means get involved because this research is crucial. But if your patient is past the moderate stage of the disease, I would think long and hard before committing.

Clinical studies take place in a variety of locations: hospitals, universities, doctors' offices or community clinics. Now, I know for a fact that if I had pulled up in front of a hospital with my dad, he would have absolutely refused to get out of the car in fear of being admitted overnight.

It's the aftereffects that cause the most hardships. It would take my father days to settle back down after a trip to an ordinary doctor's appointment.

Should you, the caregiver, consider joining a study, evaluate the terms carefully. All clinical studies have rules; there are no universal standards.

Ascertain how frequently you must attend the study and whether or not it will always be in the same location. You need to know if the patients can continue taking their present medications and how long the study will last. Side effects from new medications are possible; so watch them closely and write down anything you notice, whether you think it's vital or not. Some clinical studies pay participants for their time and travel expenses while others do not.

There are many pros and cons to consider. Since people with Alzheimer's are unable to give consent, the final decision of joining a study may fall upon the next of kin or the person who is power of attorney. A positive outcome could be that the patient involved may receive a new state-of-the-art medication years before it reaches the general public.

I would never want to discourage any caregivers from enrolling patients in a select study, but one must carefully weigh all the concerns involving people who are memory impaired. However, assisting in significant research, without which we might never find a cure for the dreaded disease of Alzheimer's, could be very satisfying.

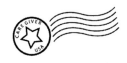

Dear Caregiver,

This poem definitely hits home:
Home is where you can be silent and still be heard ... When you can ask and find out who you are ... Where people laugh with you about yourself ... Where sorrow is divided and joy multiplied ... Where we share and love and grow.

Author Unknown

Home Sweet Home

(Nursing Homes and
Adult Living Centers)

Yes, there are people available to help, so you *can* enjoy a well-earned respite. I'm sure at some point, your Alzheimer's victim has experienced a hospital stay or perhaps even been sent to a rehabilitation facility or nursing home. You may have been approached by an on-staff social worker whose job it is to make recommendations, some of which might be worthwhile. Cautiously keep in mind that most of these referrals come from a list that was put together by their supervisors and 98 percent of the list will be compiled from "sister companies" which is an obvious prejudice. If the facility is suggesting a certain nursing home, don't be afraid to ask if they have ever set foot inside it themselves.

As much as I oppose placing Alzheimer's patients in nursing homes, a time comes when you may no longer be able to provide the care they need. But be forewarned that drastic changes will advance rapidly once you break them from their daily routine. You will likely notice the deterioration of their memory almost immediately. You might be told it's because you no longer see them on a day-to-day basis. From what I've seen, the dismantling of their routine life leaves them in a new world of confusion that's extremely difficult to overcome.

If you search hard enough, hopefully you will find a suitable facility. One of the top things you need to look at is how qualified the staff members are in dealing with dementia patients. Are they required to take a course in memory impairment? Some companies have gone from making their staff take a two-day course to only a half-hour online class. This is most irresponsible.

Learn how they supervise wandering patients, also talk to the activity director to find out what activities he or she has for the memory impaired.

This is a big one: ask if the patients have the right to continue using their regular physician. You might have to transport them to their own doctor yourself, but it should be well worth it.

Once patients become residents, they will most likely hit you with a handful of complaints. Before you go off half-cocked, investigate to see how much truth is behind these accusations. "They haven't fed me in days," is a frequent lament. Next you will likely hear them say over and over that their personal property has been stolen. It might be true, but remember how suspicious the Alzheimer's mind has become. If you feel something has to be said to the staff, say it. You are the voice for that person. If you feel the need to speak out—do it!

When visiting Alzheimer's patients, please do not keep telling yourself, "What difference does it make if I visit them. They won't remember anyway." Your being there will make a positive difference, trust me. You might be all they have left. There will be times when you walk in and they don't remember you, but the times they do will mean the world to both of you.

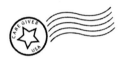

Dear Caregiver,

Walter Winchell, who is known as the invented the gossip column, said:"A real friend is one who walks in when the rest of the world walks out."

GJL

Visiting Day

(Visiting Patients)

I'm directing this segment not to the caregiver, but to relatives and friends of Alzheimer's victims.

If you're visiting with loved ones and they don't recognize who you are, this doesn't mean your time is wasted, just having someone by their side helps. Look directly into their eyes and remind them who you are. This may or may not rekindle their memory. If they still don't remember you, remember not to take it personally.

Plan your visits between late morning and early afternoon. This should be the time when they're at their best. As the day wears down, they most likely will too. You might want to bring along a photo album. Turning through the pages might inspire decent conversation. Plan an activity, something as simple as going for a walk. Fresh air always helps to stimulate the mind.

If they're speaking and not making any sense, just go with the flow. Gradually, try changing the subject if it's too bothersome for you.

You're doing the right thing by being there. People are nurtured through human contact, even if they don't always show it. Every minute you're there is worshiped.

Recently, someone shared a story with me of a man who goes to his wife's nursing home and has breakfast with her every day. She hasn't recognized him in the past five years, but what's important to him is that *he* knows who *she* is. Tough love isn't about surviving the storm, it's about learning to dance in the rain.

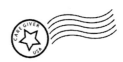

Dear Caregiver,

S. Butler said, "Friendship is like money; easier made than kept."

My father loved saying that about money. He was a generous man but also quite frugal. As his caregiver, I was privileged to observe him toss aside any feeling for money other than, "The best things in life are free."

Yes, unfortunately, money is necessary but friendship and love outweigh "all the gold in California."

Thanks, Dad. Glad we were friends.

HBM

Hidden Costs of Nursing Homes

When all other possibilities have been exhausted and the loved ones must be sheltered in a nursing home, the primary caregiver or nearest relative should be aware that the average cost of residential care in the United States is $180 per day, approximately $63,500 per year.

Even then, there are still certain expenses that will not be covered. Every facility is required to provide you with a list of items that are not part of their daily or monthly rate. These are some of the items that might not be covered:

- Laundry services
- Bedside telephone
- Hearing aids
- Eyeglasses
- Dentures
- Haircuts

Round-trip transportation for medical procedures outside the facility.

Often, there are many co-pays you will likely encounter that health insurance or Medicare might not provide: One-hundred percent coverage for certain medications, lab work, physicians' bills and physical therapy. That's just to cite a few.

Medicare seldom covers a patient's stay for more than twenty-one days, at 100 percent, and Medicaid is usually only available to low-income people. This is why it's so important to prepare financially for such eventualities as early as possible. It's not like you can just drop off loved ones and their expenses will be altogether covered. It simply doesn't work that way. In order to qualify for Medicaid, patients may have to surrender any assets they own to obtain funding for residential care.

Remember, it is difficult enough for any nursing home resident to advocate effectively for themselves. It's virtually *impossible* for Alzheimer's patients.

When residents run into problems and believe that they're not properly being cared for by the facility and feel the problem is not being resolved within the nursing home's administration, patients or their families should contact the Department of Elder Affairs and request to be appointed an *ombudsman* to look into any allegations. *Ombudsmen* are legal representatives who act as an advocate, making sure residents' rights are not being violated.

The Freedom of Information Act assures public access to any state or federal inspection reports. If the facility doesn't have them posted in a visible and accessible spot, check the results from the local Social Security office. Tour the facility yourself in advance.

Ask many questions, not only to the staff, but also current residents about the facility. Ascertain all that you can before making the final decision of placing patients there. Having loved ones admitted into any establishment is a traumatic life-changing decision. Therefore, approach this responsibility with much thought and the utmost advanced research. Meet with the center's administrator to discuss the base pay and any extra charges that may be accrued. Make sure the basic costs are in writing and don't sign *anything*, until you completely understand all financial matters entirely. There will be many papers that you'll have to endorse and they may be confusing. Take your time, read everything including the small print. Your decision needs to be the right one.

Dear Caregiver,

John Willard Marriott was an American entrepreneur and businessman who built his business from a small root beer stand into one of the world's largest hotel chains. He said: "Good timber does not grow with ease. The stronger the wind, the stronger the trees."

Being a caregiver, you will come out of this campaign with a more passionate outlook on life.

GJL

Financial Burdens of Alzheimer's

(Money Problems)

The monetary expenditure of caring for a loved one with Alzheimer's can be at least three or four times the amount of caring for an average senior adult.

Recently, I received a correspondence from a woman who has been her mother's primary caregiver for the past five years. She wrote explaining that she has to pay an outside caregiver $10-per-hour in order that she could maintain her $13-per-hour job "A little bit's better than nothing, and it gives me a chance to get some respite." Most caregivers have to give up their employment completely, bringing on the additional stress of being financially ruined. I understand her dilemma only too well as I had to cut my working hours in half, accomplishing this only with help from my beloved sister. In today's economy, how devastating is that!

Regarding pharmaceutical costs, medications currently available for Alzheimer's, which by the way may only ease the symptoms for a short length of time, are exceedingly expensive and have a Medicare Part D Plan reaching its limit so fast that you end up falling quickly into a financial hole.

- Additional costs may include as follows:
- Hiring home care
- Transforming the home into a safe haven
- Acquiring medical equipment
- Earlier admittance into a nursing home
- Incontinence products

The list goes on. These costs could bankrupt any family. The incidence of Alzheimer's is rising at an astonishing rate. It is now listed as the sixth leading cause of death and climbing. Experts have released a report that states someone in America will develop the disease every sixty-nine seconds; that's almost a person per minute and nearly a half million new cases of Alzheimer's each year.

The best advice I can offer, once again, is for the families to work together. Instead of all the burdensome costs and care falling upon any one person, it needs to be shared throughout all family members. I've found that tragedies tend to bring people together, and that is exactly what category this disease falls into—a true tragedy.

Blessed

Blessed be the awesome power that heals,
great power that fuels the very sun.
Blessed, the sculptor of the stars,
the maker of usever one.
Blessed be the wondrous power that saves
each heart that flounders on life's shoals.
Blessed, the author of the Book
that serves as lighthouse to lost souls.
Blessed are we who find the shore
where meadow lands feed hungry sheep,
and blessed are we who find ourselves,
in the Blessed Shepherd's keep.

Valerie Esker

Life Expectancy of Alzheimer's

Across the planet, there are an estimated twenty-four million people beset with Alzheimer's or some other form of dementia.

The most haunting question that runs through every caregiver or family member's mind is, "How much time does my loved one have left?"

No specific time line has been established regarding the amount of years that persons have left after their initial diagnosis. One difficulty with this research is that they are diagnosed at different stages of the disease and those affected react differently with their own unique symptoms.

According to a study executed by the University of Washington, survival from the initial diagnosis is 4.2 years for men and 5.7 years for women. (Yes it's true, women with Alzheimer's seem to live longer than men.) But I often hear from fellow caregivers and other experts that six to eight years is common. There's no way of knowing for sure exactly how long someone with Alzheimer's disease has. Some live only a few short years while others continue on, still doing well physically for a decade or better.

Basically, the older they are at the time of the diagnosis or the more severe their symptoms are, the shorter the survival period. Other factors that come into play are whether or not patients have a history of diabetes or congestive heart failure as well.

I believe that one of the most important elements in longevity is the quality of care loved ones receive while suffering from this disease. Once again, this is where a routine lifestyle becomes so essential.

When caring for your loved ones, I don't really see the need to bring up the issue of how much longer they have left. Only at the very beginning should they be appraised of what lies ahead so that their personal wishes can be heard. Nobody likes to be told they are running out of time and that they are heading into a future from which they won't be able to hide. A caregiver's goal should be to protect patients as often as possible from becoming emotionally upset.

In the twenty-first century, it is common to hear from experts that the average sixty-five-year-old can expect to live another 18.5 years. Unfortunately, in the case of those stricken with Alzheimer's, many of those years will be robbed from their life span.

For caregivers and family members, the life expectancy question is a hard one to ask, with a devastating answer even harder to swallow. But by constantly showing how much they are cherished, the path they and their caregivers are walking together can have many gratifying moments along the way.

Just do the best you can, keeping them in a routine and as comfortable as possible to the very end.

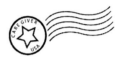

Dear Caregiver,

For every storm a rainbow
For every tear a smile.
For every care a promise
and a blessing in each trial.

Irish Blessing

HBM

Weathering the Storm

(Preparations and Evacuating)

When a natural disaster occurs, chances are, you will have no time to stop and think. Caring for a loved one afflicted with Alzheimer's during this situation will have you potentially facing two major disasters; the oncoming storm and the mass confusion of the patient.

All through the years of caring for my dad, I dealt with my share of problems, even just during typical Florida thunderstorms. When our electricity would go out for even an hour, my father would become quite alarmed. During one particular storm he became quite upset, constantly opening our refrigerator, demanding to know why the light inside would not work. Meanwhile, all we had were a couple of candles and a few flashlights which only added to his confusion.

If you find yourself in such a situation, chances are you cannot rely on other people for help as they will probably be caught up in making their own preparations.

In the event of an impending hurricane or storm, loved ones will most likely be frightened and uncooperative. The decision to evacuate may have to be made. This can prove to be exceedingly difficult for anyone who is memory impaired. Any change in routine—never mind a change in surroundings—will be very disturbing for them.

If this should happen to you plan ahead. Research where it is you may need to go. If you have a relative or friend's home to which you plan on evacuating, try to get there early enough so your loved one can be settled into his or her new environment. Prepare a checklist for a substitute caregiver listing the patient's daily habits and anything that can help to soothe him or her.

Be prepared with an evacuation kit that contains copies of the power of attorney, financial papers and also a list of doctors and medications. Have a directory consisting of family members or potential caregivers with the patient's doctors' names and locations and contact numbers. Make copies of this list and place one in your loved one's wallet or purse and the other in yours, in the event you should get separated.

Pack a bag containing medications and incontinence products if needed, along with a photo album or something you know might keep him or her at peace.

Consider pets as well. My dad was very fond of our cat and sometimes seemed to care more for the cat than himself during his time of battling this disease. I assured him that his pet's welfare would be well looked after.

Do the best to maintain a calm demeanor and have a positive conversation with your patient. Be reassuring that you're there to assist in his or her needs. Be prepared, for it will probably be necessary to repeat yourself often throughout this ordeal. It's essential that you don't get yourself into a frenzy. The calmer you appear, the less unnerved he or she will become.

When your loved one is settled down and safe, then if need be, go back and secure your home. Being followed around while attempting to board the place up will only turn into another disaster.

The best thing you can do is be prepared comfortably ahead of time. This isn't going to be an easy task; you're just going to have to wade through it.

Your local chamber of commerce will have all the information you need in the event it becomes necessary to seek out a public shelter which can best suit your needs. But keep in mind, people suffering from dementia do not perform well in noisy, crowded places.

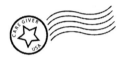

Dear Caregiver,

Have you ever been just cruising through your day when you suddenly hear lyrics from a song that stick with you for a while? Well, this Beatle song came on the radio and I heard them singing "I get by with a little help from my friends."

It just got me thinking; through a campaign of caregiving, always be grateful for all the little things people do to try to help.

GJL

Support Groups

Sharing your experiences and making new connections can make you feel better about life in general. I've found that a perfect place to accomplish this is through a support group.

One of the first things that amazed me after sitting in on my first Alzheimer's caregiver's support meeting was the number of people who still attended even after their loved ones had perished. This showed me that the caregivers that participated in these meetings were devoted to distributing their wealth of knowledge with their fellow caregivers who are now coping with the same hardships.

This type of meeting will help you feel less alone while discovering new abilities and motivation to keep up the good fight as you take on one of life's most difficult jobs.

If you are a caregiver and decide to go this route, you will discover a harmonious effect from sharing the journey you're traveling in a safe and welcome environment with people who have suffered or are suffering the same pilgrimage. Also, it is so comforting, knowing that everything that you say will always remain confidential.

Please keep in mind that this is not group counseling. If you're suffering from deep depression, you should seek professional help. Support groups are for people who share common interests and are searching for tips and advice on how to manage their own turmoil.

If you first attend a group meeting and it doesn't seem helpful, shop around. These days there are usually quite a few options for meetings in your neighborhood.

Meetings are usually scheduled once or twice a month; try to find someone to fill in for your caregiving duties. Get yourself out of the house and try out one of these support groups. They're worth investigating. I don't believe that you will be disappointed. Just the confirmation that the feelings you're experiencing are perfectly normal will have you walking out believing everything is going to be okay.

I wish that it would become mandatory for every physician who deals with Alzheimer's to attend at least one caregiver's support group meeting. I guarantee that, after that, they would start listening to caregivers a little more closely.

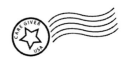

Dear Caregiver,

I loved Karen Carpenter's soulful rendition of "Bless the Beasts and the Children." Oh, how the tears would roll down my cheeks as she sang: "Give them shelter from the storm. Keep them safe, keep them warm,"

As caregivers, that is exactly what we do. Whatever "storm" your precious charge is facing, just do your best to shelter them.

You are their light in the darkness.

HBM

Elder Abuse

The Senate Special Committee on Aging estimates that as many as five million Americans may be victims of elder abuse every year.

It is not unusual for caregivers to verbally lash out at their patients due to exhaustion or frustration. Some may not consider this to be an act of abuse. But verbal abuse is labeled as emotional or psychological abuse. This act is defined as "inflicting mental pain or distress from verbal mistreatment."

Sadly, I found myself occasionally shouting at my father after being tormented with the same questions over and over again, sometimes as many as fifty times! If this should happen to you and you feel yourself beginning to reach the boiling point, step outside, get some fresh air and kick some dirt around if you have to. It's bad enough that it elevated to that point. Never let it escalate any further. These are significant signs of stress and the fact that you need a break.

The next step, right around the corner, could be physical abuse. This could include the following actions: pushing, shaking or even depriving patients of their basic needs such as withholding medications or overmedicating them. Also included on that list should be physical punishment or restraint.

If you suspect this is happening to someone you know, look for red flags, including the caregiver suddenly refusing to allow visitors, or possibly a change in the patient's behavior when the abuser comes near.

A gentleman, and I use that term loosely, told me that he once threw a hot bowl of soup on the man he was caring for. "The man kept claiming someone stole his soup at least twenty times while I was still heating it up for him. *It just happened.*"

Alzheimer's patients or those who suffer from any kind of dementia are twice as vulnerable and the signs are more difficult to distinguish. One reason is that they never tell the same story twice.

If you believe the abuse to be sexual, always investigate any allegations further. Signs of sexual abuse are not as apparent, so take whatever you're being told seriously.

Another common type of abuse is financial. The disappearance or concealment of funds, property or assets accounts for 40 percent of all abuse cases.

Neglect, another form of abuse, comes from depriving patients of their personal needs. This could include failing to supply proper clothing, shoes that do not fit correctly, or even no shoes at all. Patients' clothing must also be appropriate to weather changes—coats and gloves for winter, shorts for summer.

Abandonment is leaving them alone when you know that they need constant supervision.

The laws on elder abuse vary across state lines, but legislators in all fifty states have passed some form of prevention laws.

The National Elder Abuse Incidence Study reported that there has been an increase in elder abuse of 150 percent in a ten-year span.

These senior citizens are fragile and vulnerable. If they weren't, they would not be in need of a caregiver. Some patients won't speak up for themselves because they are afraid it might make matters worse. The fear of who will be taking care of them next keeps them quiet.

If you suspect you know of a defenseless senior who is being abused, please look into the situation. There could be an actual risk of death involved here. You can contact the Department of Elder Affairs about your concerns.

Caregivers being over-stressed is the number one cause of elder abuse. When you feel the pressure starting to build, find a way to get some respite. Call a friend or a family member. Everyone needs a break.

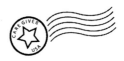

Dear Caregiver,

Ralph Waldo Emerson, an American lecturer, essayist and poet wrote this truthful statement: "It is one of the most beautiful compensations of life that no man can sincerely try to help another without helping himself."

GJL

Home Alone

(Living Alone with Dementia)

There are an overwhelming number of elderly people living alone while suffering from some form of dementia. The truth is we will never get an accurate head count since so many senior citizens live under the radar, alone, trying to fend for themselves. Sadly, even some of their own family members ignore the situation until they become seriously ill or injured.

The act of being a "Good Samaritan" has almost faded away these days. With times being as tough as they are and unemployment reaching such a high percentage, most families are struggling to keep their *own* household from collapsing.

Many of today's generation have never developed a concern for their senior neighbors, and atrociously, there are some families that just don't seem to care about what happens to their relatives. Regrettably, it often takes a tragic occurrence to force someone to take notice.

Sometimes hospitalization becomes a blessing for these lonely people as that's when most companionless dementia patients will finally at long last receive a diagnosis.

Dehydration or accidental overmedication is the most common cause for a trip to the emergency room, which later may involve a home health agency providing some overdue supervision for these patients. This could possibly lead to a court decision pertaining to their future.

The progression of Alzheimer's or other dementia-related diseases can advance rapidly. This leaves patients who are living alone running out of time faster than they had anticipated.

It is essential that we pay close attention to our senior citizens, whether in our neighborhood, church, or even in the grocery store. Look for signs of weight loss, a dwindling social life, stacks of unopened mail, or anything you might think that is out of their norm.

That "senior moment mentality" needs to become a chapter of our past. Questions and concerns should be the present and future. It's better to be apprehensive and stick our noses in then to ignore the situation all together until something critical finally happens.

If these people have family, by all means contact them. Ask the senior you're concerned about questions like, "When was the last time you've been to the doctor? Have you talked to your family lately? Where do your children live? Do you need a ride to the grocery store?" Casually try to find out any contact numbers without offending them. Don't be afraid of getting involved. You could possibly be saving their lives.

Being a "Good Samaritan" is admirable. Helping someone in trouble or distress is something to be proud of.

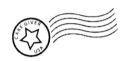

Dear Caregiver,

Thomas Jefferson, the third president of United States of America, once said: "When angry, count ten before you speak; if very angry, count a hundred."

Great advice. But, as a caregiver, hopefully you will be able to find enough time to count that high.

GJL

When They Say, "I Want to Go Home!"

Whether it's relatives, friends, nursing staff or anyone caring for those afflicted with Alzheimer's or dementia, they have heard or will inevitably hear the patients say, "I want to go home!"

Patients may even pack their bags, piling them at the front door, waiting to leave. This may happen even though they are still living in their own residence of thirty-some years.

My father would constantly ask me, "Why can't I go home? My mother is going to be awfully worried about me." This is a perfect example of a need for redirection, a caregiver's best tool of defense. For example, I would assure my dad that everything was going to be okay. "I just talked to your mother an hour ago. She knows that you'll be spending the night here so why don't you play some cards until dinner is ready?"

Just go with the flow. Obviously, they're already confused. Try to avoid making matters any worse.

Hearing the statement "I want to go home" should be taken as a potential forewarning that wandering may be in the near future. Be nonchalant but pay close attention to your loved one until you feel confident that he or she has moved on to fresh and more pleasant thoughts.

I'm directing this advice to everyone who is involved in the care of the memory impaired. This includes nursing home employees, family members, etc. This is a situation where patients can easily become lost and possibly seriously hurt.

Some may find this a bit comical, but there is a nursing home in Germany which built an exact replica of a bus stop in front of their facility. Their average patients suffer from having no short-term memory. But the long-term memory may still recall the colors of the bus sign and that waiting there means they're soon going home. The staff then gently approaches the confused patients, informing them that the bus won't be along until later in the day and then kindly invites them inside for a cup of coffee while waiting. Usually, by the time the cup's empty, the patients have completely forgotten what they were waiting for. If this keeps them from running off and getting hurt, I would call this well-intended ruse a success.

The fact that patients are unable to recognize their own surroundings makes things extremely frightening for them. They may wish that they were back in the comfort of their own home, even if they already are.

When they are saying the word "home," their definition could mean many different things. They could simply be trying to tell you they wish things would go back to the way they were.

Once again, casual redirection of an Alzheimer's patients' thoughts is something every caregiver needs to master.

Age and Transition

I weep, because you pale before my eyes,
a shadow of the father I recall
when I felt younger than my grandson's cries
of jubilation, "Nana, catch the ball!"
I hide my fear of entering this phase,
transition of the parent and the child.
I pause, then blindly stumble through the haze,
uncertainly, a monster, dark and wild.
I ask, "Feel better? You look good." (Not true.)
We talk about the weather, news events.
We waste the moments when we have so few
and brevity of life itself presents
its own distortions.
Take my hand today.
Though I'm the child, this time I'll lead the way.

Gail Teachworth

Suicide—A Silent Turning Point

Nothing devastates a family like the loss of a loved one through suicide. It is such an incomprehensible tragedy; it leaves everyone speechless, without ever having any answers.

With senior adult couples the rate of homicide-suicide increases 50 percent higher than younger adults. For those who suffer from Alzheimer's, the so-called caregiver-dependent homicide-suicides make up a large percentage of senior deaths. When a couple who has been married for a long period of time becomes totally dependent upon one another and one or both become irreversibly ill, homicide-suicide may appear to be the only answer. Periods of deep depression may trigger feelings of utter hopelessness, especially on the part of the husband who feels helpless in realizing he can no longer fulfill what deems to be his husbandly duties. This usually has him initiating the act. Do not interpret this as a suicide pact; this is an act of "desperation" and "hopelessness."

One caregiver resource report showed nearly 60 percent of caregivers experience clinical signs of depression and 40 percent of former caregivers have mild-to-severe depression which can last up to three years after the patient has died.

Family members and friends need to watch for signs that could lead to thoughts of attempting suicide.

Some years ago my brother took his own life. There were signs scattered all around me, none of which ever came to mind until it was too late. There is a window of opportunity for intervention in almost all these suicidal situations. Close friends and family members just have to be alert enough to notice them.

My brother, who was a nurse, once told me, "I can handle any part of the physical illness of the patient, but I simply cannot deal with the mental illness." I am not suggesting my father's Alzheimer's was the cause of my brother's suicide; our insufferable family problem now is that we will never know. I can honestly say that I was so angry at my brother, it stopped me from properly grieving.

Beware of any sudden changes in caregivers' behaviors. If they start giving away their prized possessions, crying for no reason, experiencing insomnia, becoming isolated from social interaction, putting their final affairs in order or voicing feeling of helplessness, these are just a few of the forewarning signs.

Many people do not realize the extraordinary circumstances connected with a suicide. For example, it became difficult for my family to make plans for a funeral. The medical examiner wouldn't release my brother's body for cremation until all forensic tests came back without any complications. This took almost a month during which my mother was devastated. There was no closure for our family and I suspect there might never be any. It took almost two months before I received a death certificate.

Families need to pay close attention to their loved ones, especially senior members, as the incidence of Alzheimer's and, often, accompanying suicides is rising to astonishing levels.

We all hope that a cure for Alzheimer's will be discovered, but until that time, we're just going to have to watch each other's backs. Suicide can become a silent turning point that changes a family forever.

Moments of Silence

Time takes care of little things
with quiet moments of laughter
to help us overcome our loss
and bring us peace thereafter.

Let's share our friendship, love and peace
by overcoming sadness
that brings us down and lays us low
until we find the gladness.

Replace it by healthy thoughts
to help us on our way
because we know that surely time
will take us all someday.

All their needs God will provide
while tucked in His wings of care
golden angels guide our steps
until the time we meet them there.

Esther Marie Latz

Final Countdown

(Last Minute Decisions and Death)

There are diverse opinions about what happens to a patient when Alzheimer's wins and the victim finally loses.

The actual cause of death might be the following:

· Malnutrition
· Dehydration
· Pneumonia
· Infection

These are just to name a few.

I believe malnutrition is the most relentless of villains. While in the last stage of Alzheimer's, getting the patient to eat is one of the hardest struggles.

Difficult decisions must be made during these times. Most likely, caregivers will ask themselves if they're being selfish by not permitting a life to end. Should they allow the ravaged to tranquilly slip away or should they pursue extreme measures, only prolonging the beloved's breathing? I don't believe there's a right or wrong answer to this dilemma. This is one of the reasons I admire Hospice organizations; they provide the peace of knowing your loved one is leaving painlessly.

Finally, the real cause of death, "Alzheimer's," is finally being recognized and now placed on death certificates. This way the world can accurately be made aware of the astronomical number of people put to death at Alzheimer's Guillotine yearly—roughly twenty-five million worldwide are afflicted, awaiting the blade.

Alzheimer's is a terminal illness. It is time for this fact to be universally acknowledged. I rarely talk to anyone these days who doesn't have a family member whose life has been stolen or devoured by this demon.

Alzheimer's is a death sentence of the mind. Thus, the mind dies before the body, leaving that pilotless tenement of anatomy fighting without a chance. My goal is to educate as many people as possible about the devastation of this disease. Knowledge is power and a crusade of great power just might win against this murderous abomination.

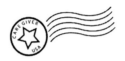

Dear Caregiver,

Buddhist Philosopher and Peace builder Daisaku Ikeda once said:"A person, who no matter how desperate the situation, gives others hope, is a true leader."

As a primary caregiver, you will learn to become a true leader.

GJL

The Long Good–bye

Just when a person's memory really begins to matter most in life, this cruel and heartless disease comes along, disrupting everything and everyone that is close.

The fact is that Alzheimer's is an irreversible disease and, unacceptably, has no known cure. It slowly steals the victim's mind, leaving a long trail of broken-down, worn-out family members and caregivers behind.

Everything comes with a price. The average American's life expectancy has increased dramatically over the last one hundred years, expediting the numbers of those plagued with Alzheimer's, making it a drastic price to pay.

There appears to be a sense of shame associated with this disease. Notoriety seems to be given to celebrity-driven causes such as breast cancer, heart disease, diabetes, etc. I'm not trying to place the importance of one fatal disease in front of the other. But, for example, a professional sport such as Major League Baseball uses Mother's Day as an opportunity to have ballplayers swinging pink bats or running in pink shoes for breast cancer awareness. Alzheimer's, on the other hand, seems to be kept lingering completely outside the ballpark.

The disability of being mentally impaired has been swept under the rug for hundreds of years. "Ol' Uncle Charlie has been very confused lately, so we decided to let him live in the cabin on the backside of the property." This attitude has stolen the attention and devotion away from this mind-devouring disease that it truly demands. Even as Alzheimer's continues to climb the scale to one of top leading causes of death, it still seems to remain stagnant on the priority list of lobbyist and politicians.

There is nothing prejudiced about this disease: creed, culture, gender, rich or poor; it will strike down anyone, taking along family members and caregivers along the way. It simply does not care!

Usually, most caregivers are a husband or wife, son or daughter that loves the patient dearly. They constantly feel that they have to give the best possible care to ensure their loved one's well-being. And sadly, it's the family who witnesses the patient slowly fading away, which has prompted many to use the sobriquet of "The Long Good-bye" for this disease. Having experienced this personally, I couldn't agree more.

At the very end, Hospice kept telling me my father wouldn't make it through the day but then found it necessary to repeat themselves fourteen days in a row. The ups and downs of this duration were mentally and physically exhausting. By the time my father passed, I barely knew my own name. My sister and I took shifts sleeping; if you could call it that. The rest of this precious time was spent tending to Dad and watching him wither away to the point where we could hardly recognize him.

This is a period of time that I like to call the "waiting room." I was afraid to leave the house for a five-minute trip to go to the store, because I didn't want to forego being with my dad for his final breath.

It came to a point where I felt like I had split personalities. There was one half of me praying that his Maker would hurry up and just take him and stop his suffering. This brings on a tidal wave of guilt. Well, let me tell you something; everyone feels this at one time or another, it's a natural reaction. Don't torment yourself over this.

The other half was pleading for him not to go! Somewhere inside myself, I believed that there was still a glimpse of hope and he would sit up and make a miraculous recovery. My heart was being torn in two different directions.

Please take my advice and don't go through this alone. Having someone with you to initiate a conversation or even cry with you is a blessing. Talk about the happy times you shared with your loved one. The fact that you have someone there gives you a chance to step outside for a minute and breathe in some fresh air. Trust me, it will be immeasurably comforting.

I personally know how difficult it is making phone call after phone call, informing family and friends that the end has now finally come. Try not to do everything yourself. Ask for help. It's nearly impossible to think straight at a time like this. It's in times like these that a family needs to pull together and lend each other support.

I don't believe those left behind ever get over losing a loved one. Somehow, we just learn to accept it.

Is Father Really Gone?

He left me with his memories
his sayings we love to hear.
He forgot to take our time together
and the sound of my name, so clear.

He left me the mementoes he loved
his pictures on the wall.
He forgot the glass of wine he drank
since I was very small.

He left behind his pipe and chair
his favorite knife to carve.
His hat on the rack, his glasses and cane
how to cook, so we never starve.

My mind knows of all his strengths
as if written on my heart,
and every time I think of him
his words do not depart.

He left his wish to continue his name,
the stories he told were not rumor.
His genuine emanating laughter
his special sense of humor.

Esther Marie Latz

After the Loss

It's difficult to find words that adequately express the deep and personal emotions one experiences after the death of a loved one.

I'm not sure if I will ever get over the loss of my father. I guess I am just hoping to get used to it. When coping with a death, one will likely go through a myriad of emotions: sadness, fear, shock, confusion, anger, guilt, exhaustion, a sense of being cheated, and even an unpleasant emptiness. Every time I feel as if I am moving on, a wave of overwhelming sorrow swells up inside of me.

I believe the best thing I did was to start remodeling the inside of my home. I chose bright and bold colors. I needed to put some life back into the house in order to keep my mind from wandering and grieving. Although the work took me weeks longer than I estimated, just keeping busy proved to be very therapeutic.

Having cared for my father for so many years, it felt as if my body had almost gone into shock when I fully realized that all my responsibilities had been lifted.

Days immediately after his passing, I was completely occupied in making final arrangements. These
tasks were mentally difficult, but it felt as if I was still
just carrying out my caregiving duties. Then it was like
a switch had suddenly been turned off. I had been
so used to Hospice constantly coming and going, always having some presence in the house, when all of
a sudden—BAM! I was all by myself. The only way I
can describe it is that I felt hollow, as if I was living in
a void.

Everyone grieves differently. My sister, for instance,
built a beautiful memorial garden in her backyard.
Myself, I write, although the first couple of weeks I
wasn't ready to put anything down on paper. Once I
resumed writing, it was as if I finally exhaled.

If the painful yearning for your loved one doesn't
seem to begin dissolving with time, it might be helpful to seek out a support group. There is something
comforting about sharing your feelings with a group
of people who have suffered a similar tragedy.

When grieving the loss of someone close, take care
that the depression doesn't lead into something worse,
such as thoughts of suicide. Should this happen, it's
imperative that the griever seek out someone to talk
with. Just speaking of your pain and hopelessness can
relieve a tremendous sense of pressure.

Give yourself time. The yearning for a loved one
can be stronger than the depression itself. Once that
person is gone, you will miss them, even hunger for
them. Don't underestimate the power of grief. It is
one of man's strongest emotions. Sadly, one doesn't
completely realize how much the presence of a loved
one is desired until that person is taken away.

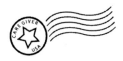

Dear Caregiver

Actress Mary Tyler Moore spoke these truthful words: "Pain nourishes your courage. You have to fail in order to practice being brave."

GJL

Aftereffects of Caregiving

Unfortunately, the chronic stress of caregiving isn't "over when it's over." After caring for someone you love for many years, you lose parts of your life that can take years to recover, if ever.

Certain side effects tend to linger on. For instance, 45 percent of caregivers go through mild-to-severe depression for up to two to three years after their loved one has passed. Many never fully recover to once again enjoy a functional social life. A caregiver must learn to accept the changes one day at a time. It's highly unlikely that they will ever look at life in the same manner after experiencing such a long emotional campaign.

An overwhelming majority will neglect his or her own health care during and after the duties are over. I know that in my case, the last sort of people I wanted to associate with were physicians or anyone else working in the medical profession. I had more than my fill of them, especially throughout the last six months of my father's life. After Dad's passing, I think it was about a year before I could bear to see a doctor for any reason.

Then there is the problem of finances. Facts show that one-third of caregivers report their income to be in the poor to near-poor range. A high percentage of caregivers that I have heard from have found it necessary to quit their jobs only to resurface in the current world of high unemployment. These people are trying to steady themselves and finally get back on their feet, while at the same time, living in a world of dismay. It's hard to describe exactly how it feels, but I can tell you that it's like living in a world of emptiness.

For almost a decade, I was devoted to the cause of caring for my dad. But when that time ended, all of a sudden it was like a floodgate was opened. It wasn't like a gentle stream flowing by; it was more like shooting the white water rapids of newly released freedom! For years prior I could barely get out to go to the grocery store and suddenly I could go wherever I wanted, whenever I wanted. But, the truth of the matter was, I didn't feel like going anywhere. Previously I had told myself that when this journey was over, I was going to treat myself to a well overdue vacation, maybe visit some old friends. But when the time came, I couldn't even get myself to leave the county!

Actually, I found myself constantly looking for something or someone else to take care of. Anybody! For instance, a sick friend with the flu, or if the cat sneezed, I was ready to rush over and hand her a tissue, a dying plant . . . it didn't matter. Truly, I finally got my fix from helping other caregivers.

There's definitely a recovery stage one must go through. So if you know any caregivers who have recently lost a loved one, give them a call. They will most likely tell you everything is fine. But the reality is that they probably need help readapting back into a social world.

Besides, that's what good friends do; help each other in times of need.

Dear Caregiver,

    I believe one of the most gifted presidential speakers we've had is Abraham Lincoln. He spoke sincerely from his heart. One of my favorite quotes from him is:"Let us have faith that right make might, and in that faith let us to the end and dare to do our duty as we understand it."

GJL

Last Full Measure

President Abraham Lincoln spoke passionately of "The last full measure of devotion" during his Gettysburg Address. His hope was that the thousands of Civil War casualties had not died in vain.

For the past decade, I witnessed my dad being whittled down to a twig.

Looking back at everything my father had endured, I've developed a heartfelt empathy for all Alzheimer's patients as well as their caregivers.

There are times when simple measures can comfort family members who also undergo an amplitude of misery from this devastating disease. For this reason, I've paid soul-stirring attention from day one, taking note how this crippling horror destroys not only its victims by robbing them of their golden years, but the lives of their surrounding loved ones. Thus, I feel compelled to share what I have learned from my experiences in hope that I can help my fellow caregivers.

When I trace my three thousand plus days of caregiving, I write about the techniques that helped relieve our greatest hardships. I found that there was no expeditious way to get through this; it was the most prolonged and painstaking road I ever marched.

Observing firsthand everything this disease stole from my family, I can only try and make sure something fruitful will grow from this. I continue to receive multiple e-mails and phone calls thanking me for the articles I write for the newspapers. A large percentage of the correspondences included the lament, "I wish I had read this while my husband was still alive." Wives, fathers, brothers, sisters and grandparents—I have heard this from them all.

Remember, knowledge is power. Former caregivers, please share helpful suggestions with your neighbor or with anyone stumbling down that rugged road of caregiving.

Until the day I die, I will preach that a regular routine is one of the most effective tactics for helping anyone suffering from memory impairment: Alzheimer's, dementia, cancer, a stroke, and any patient who suffers short-term memory loss. Routine! Please tell everyone!

Dear Caregiver,

All of us who are involved with the "Staying Afloat" venture are determined to continue in what we believe to be a vitally important exercise; the effort to keep this book circulating and finding its way into the hands of every caregiver, family member, friend, health-care provider, concerned neighbor, persons in the clergy ... anyone who has dealings with and concerns about loved ones with Alzheimer's or other dementia-related diseases. But we are urgently in need of your help! Unfortunately, we are working with a very low budget for the promotional campaign of this crucial and timely book. Please pass the word (or the book itself) on to others, especially fellow caregivers you may be in contact with at support groups.

We believe that this book will be an exceptionally helpful tool for anyone involved in caring for someone who is memory impaired.

Would you consider writing a letter to the editor of your local newspaper or favorite magazine regarding the benefits of this book? How about a posting on Facebook? If you have a caregiving-related blog, write a review or share a link to the book's Website: www.stayingafloatbook.com

This would be a valuable contribution, giving needed assistance to the millions of caregivers in the world. Many of these precious people are confused, frightened and desperately groping for answers. "Staying Afloat in a Sea of Forgetfulness" is a real "fog lifter." It is common sense caregiving at its best, laced with warm hugs, tasteful humor, and of course, a few tears.

As a concerned reader, you can help other caregivers to breathe sighs of relief as the welcome lamp of learning commences to shine brighter and brighter with the turning of each and every page.

Thank you,

GJL

INDEX